Magical Sense

Living with MS

Sue Chambers

Magical Sense – Living with M.S.
© Sue Chambers 2006

Cover design by Martin Coote, Creative Designer
Original cover artwork by the author
Page design and setting by Jaquetta Trueman, Graphic Solutions
Book text set in American Garamond 11 on 14pt
First published in 2006 by Ecademy Press

Contact:
Ecademy Press
6, Woodland Rise
Penryn
Cornwall UK
TR10 8QD
info@ecademy-press.com

Printed and Bound by Antony Rowe Ltd, Eastbourne

To my dearest sister, Judy – who had MS but they told me that she died of a brain tumour.* Her death prompted this book to be written.

> "We feel for all your sorrow
> From today and tomorrow
> Until we too depart and die
> Farewell, my friend, goodbye
>
> We'll miss you
> Your fun and your laughter
> Like the sun that always shined
>
> We're sorry for everything you went through,
> And that we couldn't help more,
> But we know you're safe and happy
> In a better place now."

I know it doesn't rhyme,
but it came from the heart.

*Actually, I found out later that it was the MS that killed her. Not fatal? Huh?

foreword

wrote this book in fits and starts from May 2001 through to 2005. The
result has been a few inconsistencies, for which I apologise. However, to
a large extent they reflect the level of uncertainty associated with the
disease I have.[1] One in particular came as a real shock to me and I've left it
as it is. To have changed it would feel like cheating to me.

I guess life isn't linear, with a steady progression. Everyone gets older,
and you do certain things at certain ages, but most people cough and
splutter, stop and start, and then re-start again – hopefully.

One more thing, without meaning to, I appear to be a diary keeper. That
is, I talk a lot to my computer,[2] and have done for years. I've used some of
my journal offerings in the text of this book. I've tried to signal this with
different margins. Please forgive any lapses of tense; it's never been one of
my strong points – ask my old boss!

[1] And others too, I expect
[2] Probably because it doesn't answer me back!

contents

Part 1

Introduction

This is a posh word for a whitter. It's really all background about me, Sue. So, hello.

A good friend asked me, "Your book, what's the opening line?" "I don't know," I replied. "I'm not even sure I'm ill enough to write it."

Well, it seemed as good as any other!

I originally meant this book to unravel some of the mysteries of MS - not really from a medical perspective, but more from a 'user friendly' point of view. When I began, I'd never even heard of the subjects in the last two parts of the book.

So that you get a sense of who's talking to you, who the 'user' is, here follows an attempt at a description of me.

- I was diagnosed with MS in the last century, back in 1985 (I try not to start describing me in terms of MS - but I assume that's why, at least in part, you're reading this book - right?)
- I was born even earlier in the last century - 1956. At the time I began writing this, that made me 45. That's when I started - I'm 47 now. And yes, it took such a long time that I've had another couple of birthdays since!
- I am a lady. (Well, that's the polite way I've heard it said.)
- Initially, my MS (because I believe it's our own illness - everyone's experience is unique) was mild enough for me to continue working for thirteen years.
- As one of four founding partners of a Market Research company my work was intense, hard and important to me.
- Work flourished, so that a colleague and myself set up a new arm of the business. He was gifted, potty and even more stubborn than I was. Am I a glutton for punishment or what?

• The new arm was about researching viewers' reactions to television - it was too interesting and, since I was Managing Director, I was too proud and stubborn to stop

Being Diagnosed With MS

Going back a bit, as I mentioned before, I was diagnosed with MS in 1985. It began on a hideous 'learn to ride' holiday – which had, by definition, horses involved. It was four days of torment – mucking out, grooming and feeding the most obstinate of beasts – all of whom were cannier than we were and could spot a virgin beginner from several miles away.

Anyway, the less said about that the better[1]. I came back with my right hand thumb alternating between numbness and violent pins and needles. Sometimes it felt as though someone had plugged my hand into an electric socket[2] – impulses were crashing up and down my hand, and arm sometimes.

Anyway, we had just got married and were feeling parent minded. So, I thought I'd better go and sort out these weird feelings, which had migrated across to the other hand. So I went off to see my GP.

I have been exceptionally fortunate with my doctors. Actually I've re-read this and realise it's not true – oh, how we forget[3]. My original GP, when this story started, was a very likeable man who we had been with for a couple of years – well, I have to admit it, quite a good looking man actually[4], as well as gentle and kind. He listened to my horse story and then sent me for carpal tunnel syndrome tests. I never did understand these – something to do with electrical signals passing up your arm? I never took the trouble to find out because, as it turned out, it wasn't that.

Next stop then. Maybe the cause was a trapped nerve in my neck? So off I went to the local hospital for X-rays, uneventful. Although it's amazing really, if you think about it – not so long ago in the history of time it would have been magical, maybe demonic even, to be able to see inside your skin. But now it's routine and radiologists are safe in their beds at night. The miracles of the NHS! I digress; it wasn't a trapped nerve either.

---

[1] Except that we did escape from the riding school to the local pub where I ordered white wine. There was much scuttling under the bar, and then the barman majestically reappeared with a glass of white wine adorned with a cocktail stick upon which he had skewered two cocktail cherries. Umm, wine cocktail...the most glorious glass of Chardonnay just doesn't quite taste the same anymore....

[2] I actually did that once – the electrician was round disconnecting my wall lights – he hadn't got as far round the room as I thought he had. Wham, across the room I flew, with tingling MS fingers.

[3] Once my first GP emigrated (see the effect I have?) I went through a couple of troublesome souls who passed for doctors as well as a good one. One GP was so difficult to communicate with that I wrote to the Family Practitioners' Board and asked to go on the books of a different doctor. That turned out to be such a good idea and found me our really good current doctor.

[4] Although, not as good looking as our dentist. A young Omar Sharif – "I'm sorry, you need another filling..." Oh, please!

My GP got a bit more serious now, "I'm afraid you may need to think about it being multiple sclerosis." He was gentle; he said it softly.

I didn't ask any more about it – he didn't want to go into it in case it wasn't - and neither did I. So we mumbled through the idea of me going to The National Hospital for Nervous Diseases in Queen's Square, London. My husband came with me for the first appointment. I remember sitting in the waiting room listening to the matron talking to a guy in his twenties. He was slumped over and had his head in his hands. From what she was saying, he had just been diagnosed with MS. I remember she suggested that he got in touch with the MS society, since he could get some help and support there. My reaction was that I would avoid this society, I didn't want to spend time with other people with MS – I thought it would only depress me and make me feel worse. This was nothing to do with the society – I didn't know anything about it. It was much more to do with me – I know I'm a very suggestible person. If I knew about certain symptoms, I could bet my bottom dollar that I would develop them at some point. I thought I would stay healthier if I didn't know much about it. Burying my head in the sand? Certainly I was. Maybe I was too scared to find out?

Thinking about it, if I'm honest, I'm still scared of MS now, nearly twenty years on.

At the appointment, it was suggested that I be booked in for a week of tests. The night before I went, I lay in our garden. I was on my back, looking at the stars. I was petrified. We hadn't told anyone – it was all between my husband Alan and me. Most notably I didn't tell my Mum and Dad – they would be so worried and my Mum would feel SO guilty. No, we had to deal with this, whatever it was, by ourselves. The thing that frightened me most was that I might have a brain tumour. It just seemed so fatal and beyond hope.

Oops, sorry, I need to stop writing for a while now. I've just realised a new connection – that I was then, most afraid of the thing that, later on, I was told my sister died of – a brain tumour.

I've slept on it. So next day, back again. I thought that writing it all down would be therapeutic. I just forgot the painful side of it. It's always been an interesting puzzle to me why psychoanalysts, ever since Freud, believe so fervently that you have to go back a fair way into the past in order to mend the present. Concentrating on the 'now' can be so much more useful, although I guess unravelling the past can help explain current behaviour and feelings. But oh, your heart can hurt in the process, can't it?

To continue with the story of my original diagnosis, we set off early (unusual for us) in the morning, following my cogitation in the back garden.

The National Hospital for Nervous Diseases takes up most of one side of Queen's Square. I don't know much about it, except for the experience I went through. The doctors and nurses were nothing but kind and helpful but the whole endeavour sent me reeling back into my own world. I guess that's right – no one should stay in the world of the sick if they can help it.

There were some in my ward who couldn't help it, poor souls. I was in a ward that was alien to me. One patient was brain-damaged and literally vegetable-like. She was in a cot in the corner by the door – very significant according to the cognoscenti. Well, one morning, she wasn't there. It's true.

Another lady, in the opposite corner by the door, had MS we were told. She couldn't walk when she came in and two nurses, one each side of her, shouted at her to put one foot forward, and then the other. Going to the loo was a slow forced march for her. It only happened a few times a day. I'm not surprised. She must have saved it up, using the evaporating force of embarrassment. She got very upset and cross at the world, especially at herself, I think. She was on a drip for a while but was feeling a bit better when I left. I never summoned up the courage to talk to her. I was too frightened. I simply did not dare to in case I bothered her, or learnt things about MS that I didn't want to know. What an isolating thing illness can be.

There was another woman in the bed opposite me who kept falling out of bed. I never worked out why.

Next to her was an epileptic. She seemed very frightened at times – but at least the nurses and not knockout drugs calmed her down. One of my cousins is epileptic. I remember spending hours in her bedroom when I was little – she was older than me and told me a lot about ballet. She had pictures of ballerinas on her walls and I think she really wanted to be one. I always thought it was sad that she wasn't and that it was her epilepsy that stopped her. I expect it's pretty difficult anyway, though.

It's also dawned on me that one of my best friends at big school was epileptic – she couldn't walk past a butcher's shop without feeling strange.[5]

In the bed next to me was a really lovely lady called Jenny. She and I

[5] Maybe she was ahead of her time – many a veggie would agree with her now.

were both in with suspected MS. We became close in that short but intense time. We both sensed that one of us would come out positive – i.e. be diagnosed with MS. I didn't want it to be her. I didn't want it to be me either – but I preferred MS to a brain tumour.

In the week I was there I went through a whole variety of tests – electrical (to measure the speed[6] of my conductive sheath[7]) perceptual, eyesight, hearing and personality. The most intriguing 'test' was a MRI scan. This was back in 1985 and the Magnetic Resonance Imaging scanner was new. It was a large round tube that you were slid into on a mortuary-type roasting tin. You went inside for about 30 minutes and, since the inside was only about 6 inches away from you, it was very claustrophobic. However, you did get a panic button – that allowed you to be a bit afraid but not feel too bad since 'panicking' was obviously normal. I transported myself to the terrace of a Mediterranean villa but unfortunately the loud clanking and whirring of the MRI, reminiscent of being inside a tumble dryer, kept jolting me back to reality.

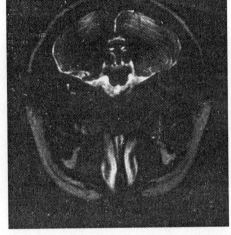

Never mind – it was an adventure, and it didn't hurt. The picture[8] is heartening in that at least there's something there. It does look more like a jellyfish though.

The hospital process began mid-week and at least I did get the weekend off. Thank God. I felt so institutionalised into the routine of The Ward. I was in danger of becoming monosyllabic and completely passive. I remember feeling totally out of control and utterly at the whim of the whole machinery of the hospital. I lost myself. Nobody seemed to know what was going to happen next, or when. I remember waiting for two days for a lumbar puncture – is that torture, or what?

The long wait for the overall verdict finally ended; the jury had been out and returned. My husband was with me at the time and we sat together on my hospital bed while a charming lady doctor told us the verdict.

---

[6] Or otherwise
[7] Note this was the cover to my nerves – nothing to do with condoms – these were pre-Aids days
[8] Don't ask me exactly what it is, all I know is that it's my brain

"You've got to remember it's not fatal," she said.

She paused.

Then she went on to explain that they couldn't be more than 90% sure, but it looked like I had MS. They had found bits of myelin sheath (remember that?) floating in my spinal fluid. The theory was that my own immune system was attacking my nervous system, leaving the bits, the debris, behind.

Back in 1985 I only knew about two forms of MS, which were described mainly in terms of how badly you had it – it was either mild or bad. Medical science didn't know that much about it, although today's knowledge about it still seems to have some way to go.

So the day of the verdict, Alan and I packed up, walked out of the hospital and fell into some chairs outside the pub on the Square. It was summertime and, amazingly for London even in this season, sunny. The recent news overwhelmed the jolly weather and the idea bubbled to the surface for me that my condition was all our business partners' fault. They had made me work too hard, not valued me enough and argued with me too much.

Unfortunately, my husband was one of my business partners and therefore got tarred with the same brush. None of it was fair really. I just needed someone, or something, to blame. However, at the time, I was quite certain it was their fault. Plus the stress, the clients, the late nights, the relentless pace, the staff problems, the book-keeping, the invoicing, the photocopier...

Once I ran out of things to blame, the shock really took over. My husband, bless him, has a great ability to make people laugh. When I was with him, it wasn't too bad. But when I was alone, the pain of feeling hard done by and victimised really hurt. Like a physical thump in the guts and literally an ache in the heart. And really, even many, many years on, there are still times when I seek out company, so I can't dwell on how hurt I feel.

That's enough of that. On a more positive note, because my MS was mild, I didn't have to explain awkward symptoms. So I just carried on in my job, told a few people at work, but not clients, and certainly not any of my family. I just did not want anyone to treat me any differently because I had MS. I suppose I thought that if they did, it would act to reinforce the idea that I had MS – not something that I wanted to dwell upon. For the same reason, I didn't join the MS society, as one of the nurses suggested. I didn't want to know about the future progression, symptoms, etc. I'm sure some people want to know but I didn't.

Psychoanalysts talk about "denial" – the idea of not accepting something unpleasant about yourself or your circumstances. Importantly, they mean this acts at an unconscious level – the denier isn't aware of it. Rather conveniently, perhaps, I've decided that this apparently negative process of denial doesn't apply to me – although I acknowledged the diagnosis and how my arm felt[9], I was, and still am, completely aware of "not making a fuss". Not only would my Mum have wholeheartedly disapproved of this[10], I also thought it would make me more ill, as though it would let the MS entrench itself into my body and soul.

People who know me say I "fight it", or that I have a positive attitude. I'm sure my Dad, were he alive, would say[11] I'm just "bloody stubborn." But he'd say it in a positive way, nonetheless.

However, Alan and I did return to the hospital for an outpatient's appointment about a month afterwards. I assume this was standard practice - to talk to patients again once the diagnosis had sunk in. We met a doctor who was new to us. He had a disability of his own. I feel awful but I can't exactly remember what it was - a bad squint, a bad leg? He gave me one of the best bits of advice I've ever had,

"Look, don't worry about it. Go away and live your life. Have your children."

So we did.

Thirteen Years On

The kind of MS that I had was clearly mild and for thirteen years it stayed that way.

During that time and after the appearance of our two kids, my interest in children and teenagers re-emerged. (I had specialised in child development for my psychology degree.) This led to me starting another arm of the business. A few others who were also certifiable and gifted joined me. While we were beginning to resemble an octopus, we forged ahead with research that specialised in listening to people aged 2-18 years.

At the time, very few market researchers included children in their repertoire. Indeed, most shuddered at the thought of being in a room with several people under 18 years old, let alone under 8. And getting these kids

---

[9] Whiz, bang, fireworks. Plus sometimes I felt that I had a tight belt around my waist – so I tied a long scarf around me. This normally happened at night – dead kinky, it looked!

[10] The fact that she never knew about my illness, not while she was alive at least, made no difference to my actions. I could still 'hear' her.

to talk about specific things? And then make sense of what they said? (If, indeed, they said anything!) Persuading clients that we could work with kids in a meaningful way was the biggest challenge of all.

I think I enjoyed it so much because it was all such a huge challenge. I drew upon my experiences and thoughts regarding kids from my degree – being the awkward cuss that I am (politely known as a rebel) - my thesis was all about trying to disprove an eminent guy called Piaget. It struck me that kids weren't as stupid and regimented as he made out and that they often acted in the way that they did because of the influence of adults. I got very close to 'proving' this in statistical terms but I didn't have a big enough sample. Not enough money, you see[12].

Nevertheless, with these thoughts as a basis, we developed various ways and means of interacting with the kids who took part in our research. I believe we developed some really good principles for conducting and interpreting our work with kids. Also, I like to think that the clients who did have faith in us and the kids we spoke with, gained some valuable insights.

I know that some people have described me as a fighter[13]. At times spearheading kids' research felt like a real battle but it was well worth it. Mainly because we were inventing the whole area as we went along, to the extent that I spoke on the radio about kids, spoke at conferences and even ran some training courses about kids' research for the Market Research Society and others.

And it felt a real let down and a shame when I became too ill to carry on. At least I trained a few other researchers who I believe have carried on the process.

Even during the time that I was still able to work, Alan helped enormously, letting me lie in at the weekend, doing the shopping and being what he called the "short-order chef." (I think that related to baked beans, bacon sandwiches and bowls of cereal). Having two fabulous kids really helped too. I say that not just because I know they'll read this but because it's true.

Then in 1998, thirteen years after I was first diagnosed, circumstances conspired to increase my stress levels to overload. I'm afraid this was all about selling the TV (and kids) research company. We sold it to some Americans, some of whom were charming but others, principally the one that stayed in the UK and 'worked' with us, were real bastards.

---

[11] With a Northern, specifically West Hartlepool, accent.
[12] Well actually, not any!
[13] I'm not sure they meant this in a positive way!

I worked harder than ever. Being 7 hours behind[14] meant that I was often in contact with them well into the night. Having a mind that never seems to stop, even when the rest of me is asleep, meant that a proper rest was, for me, elusive.

In effect, these new owners destroyed the company that we'd spent a decade building. A lot of our employees left – they couldn't stand it. The whole experience, especially not being valued, virtually destroyed me too. As a result, my body changed for the worse, and I had to completely stop work. I couldn't think, let alone concentrate, nor could I walk or generally move very well. At times, I couldn't even speak coherently. So that was the end of my career.

My GP sent me to a consultant neurologist who sent me for a MRI scan, which confirmed the diagnosis of MS. No spinal tap this time, no electrical tests and no X-rays. By this time, 1998, things had moved on and all that was required was the MRI scan. It's an amazing thing and I thought you might like to see a bit of it. I recognise the eyeballs – but beyond that...

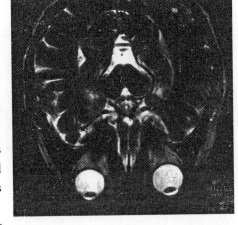

By this time, our two kids were 11 and 8. (My husband would kill me if I told you his age!)

I was desperately cross that my energy levels dropped through the floor. For example, even at home:

- If I put a load of washing on, I'd need two hours to recover.
- It took five minutes to get up a dozen stairs.
- Running up the stairs was unthinkable.
- Feed the pets? (2 dogs, 4 cats!) I despaired at the thought.
- Feed the kids (2) – impossible (enough said!)

You'll understand then, that I needed a lot of help to look after our kids and home.

---

[14] I'll restrain myself about other ways in which I thought they were "behind"

Now, as I write this in 2001[15], I still need help at home, but I'm 'with it' enough to ferry the kids around, conjure up some sort of tea and be awake between 10 a.m. and 11 p.m. That's it - being vertical the whole of that time is another matter.

Now in 2003, I still drive a manual car - driving has always been one of my passions - but my walking and balance are appalling. I need a stick all the time and going upstairs is always a two-person job. (One of them, at least, is me!) Cooking, which I loved, is beyond me most days, so tea is often a take-away!

In the last five years, most of the time life has involved trying to adjust to many, very fundamental things. The key points, in chronological order, have been trying to:

- Stop feeling guilty, since I couldn't do much.
- Stop feeling worthless, because I couldn't work anymore.

People still ask me if I miss working. In all honesty I can now say "no". I certainly don't miss the clients who, I'm sure for reasons and pressures of their own, demanded some amazing feats from us. But I do miss the kids and the teenagers that I used to talk and listen to. They were complete strangers to me and, over the course of several years, there must have been about a thousand of them, from different walks of life. I guess the trade-off is that I now have more time to spend with my own. Not so bad then – mostly.

- Somehow accept that I had MS - or at least that I had something which I had to learn to make the most of.
- Deal with people's reactions to me. This varied depending on how I was moving around. The range included:
- Me in a wheelchair on bad days or when there was travelling to do, or a lot of walking involved, like going round (and round) IKEA.
- Me holding on to the arm of an available 'balanced' person or, to be honest, occasionally a complete stranger.
- Me with a walking stick to help me balance.
- On worse days, me with both of the two options above.
- Me going along, trying to walk normally, but still noticeably limping.

- Me moving slowly, in any of the above options.
- Answer the dreaded, "Oh, what do you do?" question that you classically get asked when you're talking to someone you've never met before at a party. (Huh, I should be so lucky to get to a party!) This was especially difficult when it was a good day because I appeared 'normal'. (Well, sort of!) I mean, what do you say to try and explain that you don't do anything because you're too ill, or too low in energy, or your brain has melted? Or…? And not show the emotions that go with it all?

These were the hardest things. They can all be summed up as efforts to keep sane and moving. More about them in Part Two!

Not surprisingly perhaps, the biggest thing that happened, apart from my own MS, was my sister's.

Judy was first diagnosed in 1989. Three years after me although no one in my family knew about my MS at the time. I told her when she came out of hospital but I never told my Mum and Dad. At the time there was no need - you couldn't tell by looking at me then.

Interestingly, by then there were three kinds of MS, as reported by Judy. These were relapsing-remitting (which is the one she said she had), primary and secondary progressive MS. Neither of us liked the sound of the progressive ones, so we didn't dwell on the subject.

I tried to help Judy by talking, sharing and suggesting ideas about MS. I tried to get to see her once a week. While I think it helped her a bit, overall her approach was different to mine. Our Mum used to say that Judy "would meet the devil coming half way down the street". I'll leave you to work that one out but she certainly seemed more negative and absorbed by her MS. Although she sometimes identified with the relapsing-remitting type of MS, overall she became adamant that she had the progressive type – i.e. it was just getting worse and worse. Maybe she had secondary progressive MS?

Sometimes she seemed stable for a while, although she couldn't walk without help. Sporadically and cumulatively various parts of her would stop working and she experienced pain in varying places. Overall, this pattern stayed the same for some years – say ten or so.

Then my sister and her husband, Peter, moved home. Her two grown-up daughters had homes of their own, so there was just the two of them and the dog. They moved from a house into a bungalow – good plan, no stairs. She worried so much about the move. Well, apart from divorce, it is supposed to be one of the most stressful things you can do. So it wasn't surprising perhaps, that she deteriorated and had to go into hospital. I went to see her there and tried to joke that at least she missed the actual day of moving but it didn't stop her worrying.

A couple of weeks after the move she went to her new home for the first time.

Her decline continued. Next, she worried about her daughter's wedding the following September. She didn't want to attend in a wheelchair. Well, she was a strong-willed person - as it turned out, she didn't have to.

She died on 13th February 2001.

She went into a coma the day before and since she had made a 'living-will' (i.e. do not resuscitate) her life-support machine was turned off. It was what she wanted. She'd got to the point where she couldn't even feed herself and I think all life-processes were difficult. Overall, life had become so miserable for her that she didn't want to continue.

My bereaved brother-in-law was, bless him, at pains to reassure me that it wasn't the MS that killed her (at the time I didn't think it was fatal) - a brain tumour did. I held on to that thought very hard during the weeks following her death, especially at her funeral.

Months later, I received Judy's death certificate. I can't (don't want to?) remember exactly what it said but I showed it to my consultant neurologist. He wrote to the Coroner's Office to check on the cause of death as recorded by the post mortem. It was confirmed that she died of MS, **not** a tumour. This was my reaction at the time.

> I've just found out that my sister didn't die of a brain tumour – it was from raised inter-cranial pressure (a REALLY bad head day) as a result of acute plaques (the remains of bits of your damaged nervous tissue that your immune system has waged war on) resulting from MS. Apparently this can be clinically confused with a brain tumour.
>
> I think this is good news for her and for me. I'm really glad that there was no brain tumour that the medics failed to find. It means that I don't have to ponder any longer about whether more could have been done for her.
>
> It's good for me because I can stop being so afraid of getting a

brain tumour. I had an MRI brain scan the other day just to make sure that I didn't have a tumour and although it occurred to me, again, that it's amazing what can be seen inside you without opening you up, it's a frightening (and deafening) experience. Especially since the radiologists took me out of the scanner, gave me an injection and then put me back in again for more scans. They said they couldn't see the blood vessels properly. They were in a more jovial mood when they eventually brought me out again, so I hoped all was well. Still, you can't help but worry, can you?

But life's not that simple, is it? I thought MS wasn't fatal. Now it seems my sister died from it.

Bugger.
And where does that leave me? Well, I have to keep telling myself that she and I were very different. That the way she was and the way she died has no implications for me. If I keep saying it hard enough and long enough, I guess one day I'll believe it.

The faith comes and goes.

2

Some thoughts about living with MS, myths and maybe a bit of magic

Now there are four recognised types of MS — the three mentioned above (page 21) plus 'Benign MS'. I finally recognise myself in the fourth type because apparently this type shows little sign of disability for 10 to 15 years after the first onset of symptoms. Thereafter, disability may occasionally develop. Yeah, well, that seems to be the case for yours truly.

KEEPING SANE

Counselling

Try and keep an open mind. Personally, I think counselling is misunderstood and gets a tough time from the media. It seems fashionable now to knock it, even though its principal role is to listen and to help clients to find their own conclusions.

My GP had sent me to see a counsellor as soon as it became apparent I had to stop work. I had trouble with the idea of not working and I couldn't stop the tears, even though I thought it would only be for 6 months at the most. Maybe my GP knew better because she despatched me off to a counsellor. Being able to talk to a complete stranger, who would just listen, was invaluable. It really did help me to sort my head out — somehow talking helped my thought processes[1]. Also having someone there, just for you (albeit strictly for an hour at a time — once or twice a week) who didn't judge you, was incredibly supportive.

[1] That's why we ladies natter so much!

I still see her now, six years later. She helps me to see patterns that I live with but can't see for myself without help. I go less frequently now, say once every couple of months. I still find the outlet for my emotions very important, if I want to stay sane.

Now, Who Am I?

This was a really key question that I had to sort out in my head. It took me a long time and I'm still not sure I am entirely at peace with the outcome. I've sort of put the answer on 'hold' — I guess I'm still waiting for something to change/improve/happen, before I finally decide who I am.

The problem is complex.
What defines who you are?

— What do you do (for a living)? Back to the dreaded party question. Parties aside, in our society, our occupation seems to form a huge part of our own identity. If you stop working, a whole world of behaviour, yours and other people's, stops too. You've lost all the strokes, camaraderie, reactions, respect and, it has to be said, negative feelings, that kept reinforcing who you are. Ask anyone who has recently retired or been made redundant.

— I guess your close family and friends play a large part in defining you and, hopefully, keeping you sane. After all, they're with you more than anyone else. But, it's no surprise; living with someone with MS can be extremely hard. People have to understand, and accept that the person they thought they knew has changed. There will be some things the MS person can't do any more, some of these never mattered before but are now critical and so on.

— How do you get to know people? The context within which you meet probably sketches the outline of who you are seen to be. Maybe you have something in common which brings you together (kids, pets, train spotting?)

If you have limited energy and mobility though, the options get vastly reduced. Probably if you get ill, you can't do what you used to do, so you have to change and do what you can. Importantly, meeting new people who only knew me, as I already was, not how I used to be, was critical to me. This brings me on to the next point very neatly.

Getting Out, Doing Something New

I suspect both these things are important. I did a few things like this.

I started to go to a local shop where you could buy and paint ceramics – this felt like real therapy to me, plus I could stay there for hours. The lady who owned it was also really lovely and we became good friends. I went there for about three years and my daughter, Alice, loved it too. The outcome was that we have loads of plates, some of which are upright on stands, figures (mainly angels but also two cows and a cat!), bowls, mugs galore and a couple of candlesticks.

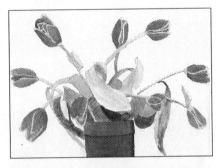

I also went to art classes for three years. They said I was shit at art at school but I'm sure that we all have the ability and maybe the need, to do art. I produced some reasonable still lifes, including naked people, as well as flowers and pots, landscapes and other watercolours, chalk drawings (try black chalk on black paper – it's wild!) and pastels.

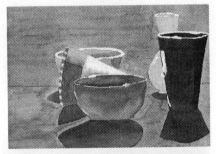

It was a long class – nearly three hours – and I had to stop eventually because my right hand wasn't working very well and had a habit of suddenly shooting out across the page. When it did that, sod's law said it was holding something that left a mark across the page. This left some interesting effects, and my art teacher, bless her soul, tried very hard to encourage me by saying it all added to my

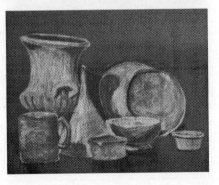

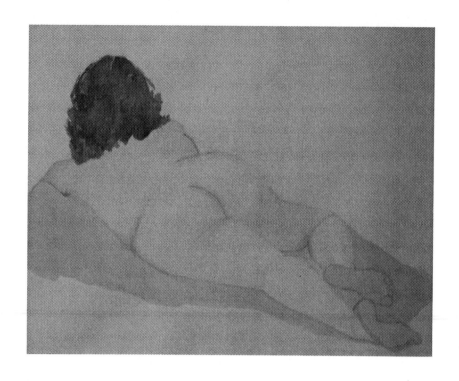

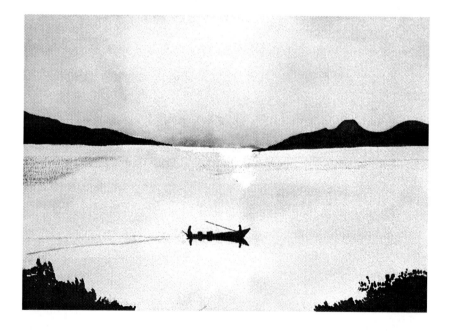

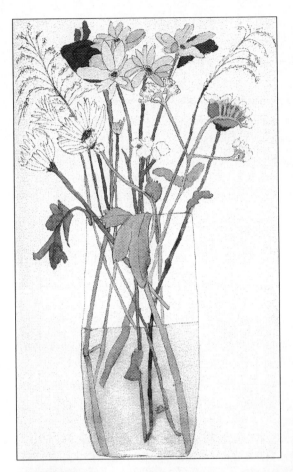

This is one of my favourites
because it shows how delicate
I can be!

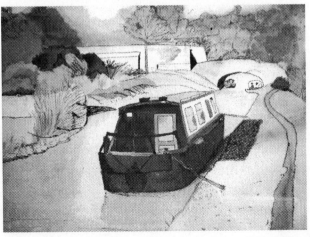

style! In the end it also became too difficult to get there, park, drag my art bag in, stay upright, concentrate, be 'arty' and get home again. There were some fabulous people there – all ten or so of us just kept going to the same class every year.

It definitely helped my sanity to get 'out'. And I want to tell you about the course I went on at my local college. Not only was it new and got me out but who knows, it might be useful one day.

I talked my way into a part-time (3 hours a week) place on a counselling course at the college around the corner from me. The course (RSA for anyone who's interested) was a beginners' course, lasting for one year. I started the course because a counsellor had helped me. I'd been off work for a year and a half when I started. We kept a journal (once a week for a year) and this is how it began:

> "Started the course and it was so extraordinary. We all met at reception, about 14 people appeared – all women, most looking very nervous. I thought someone to welcome people would have been good – the receptionist was there but really it needed a special mechanism to put people at ease. Some of us tried but I expect no one really felt it was her place.
>
> We were led to G16 in the block at the back of the car park – couldn't quite keep up with everyone but a friendly, maybe needy/nervous or considerate lady waited for me.
>
> Went for coffee. Met someone with 3 kids, – she's not sure she can manage some things – like tutorials at 9.15. Works on the phones at Childline. (An idea. Takes 4 months training though?)
>
> Someone else was very edgy and said she lacked confidence after an illness lasting a year (cancer?). She disappeared quickly at coffee time – I want to talk to her next week and share experiences. I expect it would do us both good. Later on this person mentioned wanting to be a cancer counsellor."

Overall, the counselling course was good. It taught me to really listen. I was a market researcher before MS and I thought I was really good at listening. But after this course I realised I was a mere novice listener. When I get better (that took a lot of re-writing – it started 'as if', then 'I'd really like to…'). I want to do the next two years studying that it takes to be a counsellor, and specialise in teenagers/kids.

Nevertheless, learning to listen properly has helped a lot when interacting with my kids. (They'll read this too! You agree, don't you?) Not to mention some adults.

Of course, most days I could get out – not something that my sister could always do. In her last spell in hospital I was delighted when she said she was going to try and get a motorised wheelchair. They had one on the ward she was in and she really appreciated being able to get around. It took a bit of getting used to – not going round in circles, not knocking people over, not causing traffic jams, etc!

Staying Mobile

One of the most important things to me is the ability to drive a car. From the time I had to give up work, I've been keenly aware of the fact that I could drive and 'get out' and have guarded this very strongly. I bought an inoffensive Nissan Micra in a wild bright blue and began to quite happily potter about in it. Then I noticed that me and my Micra weren't given a lot of respect on the road. To begin with, it took much longer for someone to come along who would let me out at a 'slow' junction. Also, lots of drivers would turn out in front of me. Maybe they thought that Micras were normally driven slower than some other cars?

Anyway, I'm not at all prone to road rage of any kind, but I soon got fed up with other drivers 'picking on' me and my Micra. So, I tended to drive more like I did when I was driving a car that got more respect. I tended to edge out at 'slow' junctions (as long as it was safe, I tended not to wait to be given 'the nod') and I drove a bit quicker so that people judged that it wasn't so easy to turn in front of me.

There was a time when my sight wasn't very good and I stopped driving. I have a friend with MS who lost her sight completely. Fortunately, this lasted for about 6 weeks for her and my sight was double, not lost. My normal vision also returned after about a month.

So I very gratefully returned to the road. Except that I didn't drive very far in one go. A trip into London (which took about 40 minutes and is only about 10 miles) was my limit. In my travels around the UK doing market research, many people have told me that they couldn't bear to drive around

London. I guess it depends how well you know it and what you're used to. Actually, I've been doing it since I was 17 and I love it.

However, I stopped motorway driving when my sister died, especially if I was on my own. After that, one of the best things I did was to buy a new Mini Cooper to cheer myself up. It's British racing green with a white roof. I love her. She's called Enid.

It didn't take me long to realise, though, that other drivers didn't expect someone with a walking stick to get out of the driver's seat of a Mini Cooper. I felt like putting a notice on my car explaining that I was fine sitting down, I just had balance and walking problems and just needed others to show a bit of patience!

Recently, I have not driven when my feet wouldn't move well enough or quickly enough on the pedals. I tried an automatic but it didn't help. It made me realise that the problem for me was more about the relative height of the pedals since, if there was a problem, which there wasn't most of the time, it was lifting my foot up.

Imagine my horror then, when in April 2004 I drove (at only about 10 mph) into the back of a stationary vehicle as it was queuing to get onto a mini-roundabout. It was the route to school – I knew it well. The guy I hit was in his sixties and he was understandably very cross when he first jumped out of his car and stormed round to my driver's door. I very quickly said I was sorry and that it was my fault. Ever since then he's been very kind, especially since his passenger, his son, was hurt with whiplash. Due to the injury an ambulance arrived and the police[2] came along too. Tom, who was my passenger, was brilliant – he looked after me and went to get a bottle of water for everyone.

It was all very good-natured. I think this was because the gentleman I hit, who was called, believe it or not, Mr Cooper, was so kind and forgiving. I've spoken to him on the 'phone a couple of times. His son's neck still hurts and his engagement has broken off. Mr. Cooper's car (of which he was very fond) has been declared a write-off and his shoulder and upper arm still hurt. Despite all this, he is still very nice to me and keeps reassuring me that we all make mistakes and that I should get back to driving since I haven't driven for the six weeks since the accident.

I now have it in my head that I want to have my driving evaluated by a proper[3] driving instructor. While I'm not sure what happened to cause me to go into the back of Mr. Cooper, I think my right foot slipped off the brake

[2] Who were also very kind. They took my statement and apologised when they made all the drivers take a breathalyser test – a new directive apparently.
[3] By which I mean someone who understands MS and disabled mobility issues.

onto the accelerator. (That's what's in my statement to the police). I hate the idea of not being safe on the road. What if I had hit something at a higher speed? What if it had been a pedestrian, a child? I can't bear that thought, no matter how precious being able to drive is to me.

Having spoken to a lady from MAVIS (Mobility Advice and Vehicle Information Service) I understand that you can get an adaptation for a vehicle that you can clip on and off. That kind of idea will be the one for Enid and me[4]. I phoned a 'sister' place in Welwyn Garden City, as it's nearer than MAVIS. Whatever happens, I'll have to wait a while to be 'tested', since they're very busy.

Seeing Friends

I think having friends, seeing them and making new ones became more important to me than ever once I became too ill to work. This seems obvious since my job was very social, albeit with colleagues, clients and respondents.

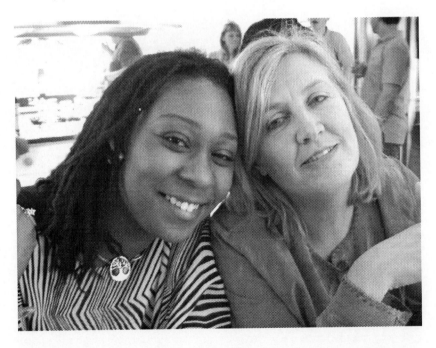

Now my friends, be they close or acquaintances, be they old or young, recent or long-established, are very important to me; this is me with Shaz who I used to work with.

---

[4] Although I can't imagine they've adapted many Mini Coopers for a "disabled" driver. Or maybe that's just my prejudice showing through.

I'm not very good in the evening anymore and can't drink much alcohol, so seeing someone around lunchtime seems to work best for me. I tend to see them on a 1-1 basis because both of us seem to get more out of the meeting that way – well I do anyway. This isn't to say that my husband and I don't socialise as a couple – we do, but less often.

I think going out and seeing people may have been one of the big differences between my sister and I. While I see friends almost every day, she spent a lot of time at home, on her own. At best, she interacted with the telly. If someone phoned her during Countdown she simply ignored the 'phone. This isn't to say she didn't have any friends – she did. The crematorium was full at her funeral, with many people that her husband didn't really know. Most of them were from the MS Society.

STRESS

Obviously this subject is huge. There are many books about coping with stress, and I have to confess I've not read many. So my thoughts are very individual – they might help, or you might spit on them!

Parenting

I found that no one could wind me up as much as my own kids. Having been at home now for several years, it's become quite clear to me that, regardless of how much I love them and miss them when they're not around, the summer school holidays nearly do me in. Nine or ten weeks of having my 'space' invaded by them and their assorted friends absolutely drains me – I can't wait for school to start again!

So, despite the 4 or 5 years of kids' research that I had done, when I must have met over 1,000 kids from all sorts of backgrounds, it transpired that sharing some genes was what really lit the blue touch paper!

Unlike the occasional adult that I'd argued with and then made a dramatic exit, I felt I couldn't leave my kids and walk out of the house. So we remained indoors, in close proximity, and the problem, whatever it was, had to be addressed. Which could be a source of more stress. But, how could I stop the process?

One of the things that I find most interesting about parenting is the thought that most of us learn it from our own mum and dad. Therefore, if any 'mistakes' are made, guess what? We repeat them.

It's so obvious but how much notice is taken of this? Do we try and help people in troubled regions, racked with prejudices, to learn a better way? No, we concentrate on the politics and expect that to filter through to the rest of the population, all of whom are trying to live daily life as best they can.

I met an Irish guy – he had been through counselling. He'd been one of 14 kids in a 3-bedroomed council house in Belfast. He talked about his 'recovery' – he said he had been very aggressive. He felt he had to accept what happened to him (was it abuse? neglect?). He didn't want to know why since what concerned him was to break the chain – to not repeat what had happened to him as he grew up. He left his family and Northern Ireland in order to avoid repeating the experience for his own children.

If the main aim is to avoid stress, then I thought that maybe I have to think afresh about what's happening? And maybe this included NOT doing what first came into my mind, since this might be based on learned behaviour which might not be appropriate to me as a parent or to my kids.

I remember listening to someone in counselling talking about 'instructing' her kids to "clean your room." It was one of her battles and it was also one of mine. From another perspective, someone else talked about memories of their parents telling them to clean their room. They took no notice either, they didn't actually think it needed cleaning. Clearly the parents and the kids may have had a different definition of 'need'.

Slowly, we learned in counselling to be more empathetic. This isn't the same as sympathetic. Empathy is about understanding another person's viewpoint, putting yourself in their shoes.

I started to talk more to my kids, especially to the one that wound me up more. I hoped that through **listening** I might understand how issues looked to him.

The listening bit is really important – true listening takes practice. It involves suspending all your own thoughts about whatever you hear, and really absorbing what you're being told.

Don't think about it and don't add in any thoughts of your own. You're not having a conversation but rather you're trying to understand the other person's point of view. You have to keep quiet yourself in order to listen properly – now is not the time for your input.

Clarification is OK, but only via repeating something the other person has already said, so that they are encouraged to tell you more. Remember that you're not doing the talking, they are. Also, be aware why you want clarification – are you being nosy, or will it really help you understand?

There's much more to counselling, but I know the above helped me to reduce the stress that could be caused without even stepping outside of the house.

I decided that I did not want to instruct my children – I couldn't deal with the conflict that would arise. I'd rather work out ways to gently persuade than to instruct which I thought would cause conflict (son) or get quiet resentment (daughter).

The result of my 'gentle persuasion' has been that the kids think for themselves and take responsibility for their own actions. Not always, of course, but some of the time. If I'm looking for positive outcomes from having MS, I hope this is one. I couldn't risk the stress that fighting/arguing with our kids might cause. I was terrified that it would make me much worse and I couldn't go through life blaming anyone else, especially my own kids, for that.

I think the process of listening began when our son, Tom, was twelve. He had been through a time when he came back from school feeling cross and acted very aggressively. This used to wind me up, I thought it was my responsibility – that I should try and calm him down and get him to stop. Of course, I didn't have to react like that. I didn't have to rise to it – i.e. let the stress take over. His feelings were his responsibility, not mine. As his mum, I wanted to try and help him feel better, but I decided that I should not take his behaviour personally.

I had help with this approach from a book[5], which I've nearly finished. It's well worth a read – I stopped because I wanted to put their suggestions into practice. This, together with proper listening, helped me accept however my kids were feeling, and let them sort out their own thoughts and reactions for themselves. (I hope.)

A case in point is the dreaded studying for exams. I can't tell you the number of times I bit my tongue, so I didn't say "have you done your ..." or other such parental things. It took a while, and some repetition, to get my husband to stop saying "dad type" things, i.e. what immediately popped into his mind from the recesses of his own childhood memories. But bless him, he did button it!

We've also sat through quite a few parents' evenings hearing how our son could do so much better, if only he tried and was more consistent. Facing Tom with that got the reaction, "but I can't be bothered". Ugh, potential murder.

But in the end it was Tom that had to decide. I think one of the most memorable parents' evenings we went to, and Tom came too, was when we spoke to his maths teacher. This charming, somewhat eccentric, older teacher told us about the trials and tribulations of Tom. How could someone get parts 1 and 2 of the question correct, and then completely lose it at part 3? His answer, which he said he had only found after giving a lot of thought to Tom, was that Tom might be insane. He appeared to be quite serious, if good-humoured about it.

Clearly, he wasn't too worried about Tom's sanity since a year later he took him and a few other pupils to the Southern tip of India, to teach local

[5] The Heart of Parenting by John Gottman with Joan Declaire

kids English pronunciation. Tom absolutely adored it and maybe a bit of insanity helped! Although nobody looks mad in this picture:

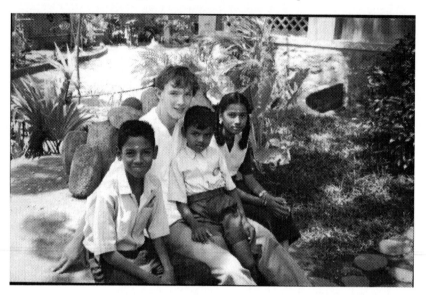

Guess what Tom got for his maths GCSE? 'A' – his teacher and his Dad (who helped him) were ever so pleased. He did pretty well overall in his exams. Anyway, well done Tom and thank goodness for that – I would have looked a right twit, wouldn't I, if my master plan had gone wrong?

Obviously, time moves on, and since writing the above Tom has taken his A/S's and now does his A2 exams this summer. So, my master plan is under scrutiny again. Except this time, it feels more crucial (he needs 2A's and a B to get to Newcastle University to do English) and Tom feels under more pressure than ever. However – I can't work it out – he seems to be doing less work than ever and yet he says himself that he needs to do some. Getting distracted seems to be one of his problems, either by friends or X-box games. His rationale for these 'distractions' appears to be that he needs a break from studying – yes, well – what studying? A friend in the same position tells me that this is normal! We also decided that this pattern wasn't how we remembered our A levels. Clearly, things have changed – the introduction of A/S, which has resulted in 3 consecutive years of exams, either means they have learnt more along the way[6], or they've got 'exam fatigue'![7]

So, I don't know. Maybe I'll just resort to my long held belief that being positive can only help.

[6] And hence they can avoid the mad cramming of two years work, that my contemporaries and I did for our A level exams.
[7] At least we had a year's rest between O and A levels.

Reinforcing 'good' behaviour once it's been done, rather than punishing 'bad' behaviour, must be the way. 'Bad' can't be ignored, but distractions can help diffuse otherwise confrontational situations. This seems particularly the case for many children (and adults, come to think of it) plus furry animals.

After all, punishment is still attention – so if it's attention that the protagonist is after, then punishment will do fine. So, if doing something wrong/bad is how attention was obtained before, then, if more attention is sought, then the same behaviour will re-occur. Rewarding 'good' behaviour with attention of some kind will also result in that behaviour being repeated – except this way you work towards behaviour that you like rather than being driven crazy by things happening that incense you.

Although I came across this simple idea during my degree, it has repeatedly come back to me and has been very helpful in dealing with all kinds of people – clients, my children, other people's children and dogs.

However, back to Tom and his A2's. The problem here is that I'm struggling to find good behaviour (i.e. studying of some kind) to reinforce.

Distraction – that's the key!

Next, Alice! She starts the Exam treadmill next year, 2006. However, she, bless her, has shown signs of planning ahead and working harder already. It is an accepted norm (in some quarters at least) that girls are more conscientious than boys. Being a girl (once!) I would agree with that!

I couldn't resist this picture. It was taken on holiday in 2004 (Alice

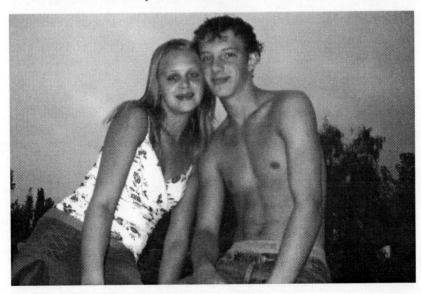

14, Tom 17). And I guess at the end of the
day, they're really fabulous people (being their
mum, I'm bound to think that) and that's what
really matters.

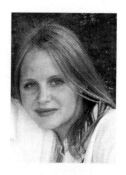

One more indulgence while I'm here. Since
there's another photo of Tom in the book, it only
seemed right that there should be another of Alice
too. Trouble is that she and I chose different shots, so
after playing around with options on the computer,
we settled at one picture each. I'm sure you can work
out who chose which!

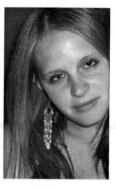

Partners

I thought writing about children was hard
enough, but this is harder!

Again, we are 'told' how to live with our partner.
Not entirely, of course, but culture is important. You
don't need me to tell you about your own culture,
but if something stresses you about your other half, it
might help to work out where the behaviour, or your reaction to it, comes
from.

For example, an Indian lady I knew talked about her husband telling
her not to defy her mother-in-law. Culturally, she expected this, but it still
stressed her out. She thought that maybe if she learnt to 'compartmentalise'
her feelings about this, she could contain them to apply only to the things
her mother-in-law actually commented upon. Then she could stop neg-
atively applying them in her head to everything – i.e. thinking to herself, "I
bet she would say…" That at least reduced her stress.

Think of patterns – what happens that winds you up? How do you react
to certain circumstances? For example, it drives me crazy if my husband
reads when we're together. I wouldn't mind a bit of communal reading, but
not when I want to talk. What's the matter with him? Isn't he telepathic?
Do I get indignant or what?

One day we talked of patterns at counselling. I mentioned my husband's
reading, and out it came – Alan had told me that his father did it, e.g.
Alan's Dad read while Eva, Alan's Mum, talked. He even used to grunt
when Eva took breath. This encouraged her to keep going! This realisation

about familial history didn't make me try and stop my husband (?) but I was more tolerant of his reading. Not very tolerant, just more.

One book that Alan read, that surprisingly he found interesting, was *Manhood* by Steve Biddulph. I saw Steve speak at a NSPCC conference. Being Australian and a Dad himself meant he had a particular view of fatherhood. While there were some traces of the Aussie XXXX humour, it was also very sensitive and loving.

Work

As I mentioned earlier, I haven't worked for many years now. I've kept this section in though just to reiterate that I suspect that listening, empathising, being decisive and aware of the patterns involved in people's working life and behaviour, could help.

I was personnel manager at work for a long time, mostly because no one else would do it. However, I'd be lying if I said I didn't enjoy it, I did. Although people came and went – I could hire them and fire them – many stayed. However, the basic problems tended to remain – they just ebbed and flowed. It also became clear to me that nobody is 'normal'.

Across the 16 years that looking after our 'employees' and their troubles was part of my working day, all kinds of things emerged. We had people who lied, who stole, who were alcoholics and those that simply pushed their luck too far.

Apart from the thieving, most of the time I tended to talk these problems through. Firstly with the person in the 'spotlight' and then to the people they worked with, including those 'above' them and those 'below'.

Sometimes the original problem wasn't work based. One person's spouse was clinically diagnosed 'insane'. It was a mixture of getting this person to talk about it more openly and get more support from the rest of us, plus the person realising that there was still a job to do and we needed the person to do it. In fact, apart from the occasional person who simply couldn't do the job,[8] most of the problems originated outside of work. Even low self-confidence could be seen as an existing personality trait, although I believe that work-mates can help here, if they become aware of it. Obviously, there were some personality clashes, although not many. A bit of shuffling sometimes took care of that. Otherwise someone had to go.

One of the hardest things to mediate was trying to persuade co-workers

---

[8] I blame the hirer for this – everyone else did!

to give someone a 'second chance'. As we all know, once somewhere/someone has a bad image, it's very hard to shift it. There were quite a few instances where someone had been stupid, selfish or misinformed and needed to 'turn over a new leaf'. Sometimes people were willing to give someone another chance, sometimes they weren't.

So, what happened about the thieving? Having tried a variety of tactics[9] to catch the thief, I gave up and let the police deal with it. They came into the office and started interviewing the staff and very quickly got a confession. We were all stunned by who it was. This person had worked with us, happily, for 3 or 4 years. Since some of the stuff that had gone missing was personal, it hit everyone even harder.

Obviously, work can be a big source of stress. But, maybe there are ways to reduce it for yourself – either environmentally, psychologically or practically. I suspect the medical profession is only just starting to under-stand what stress does to us, but there are many therapies that might help support you through unavoidable stress. I know I didn't take it seriously enough, and look what my body did to me!

I guess there is a conundrum here. You either put yourself on the 'at risk' register by putting your heart and soul into something, making you very vulnerable, or you steer clear of work stress and keep fit and healthy. The latter way hopefully you stay off the 'register', but do people start to call you 'lazy' and/or say you're not committed enough? Do they start to threaten your job?

There must be a balance here that I guess some people have sussed. A better understanding of stress and the damage it can do must help. At the same time, maybe we should examine the 'protestant work ethic' and understand what it is that drives us on?

---

[9] Marked money, surveillance shifts, a mental diary of where everyone was so we could narrow down who had the opportunity, and publicly informing everyone of what was going on (to try and shame the culprit or get some kind of reaction).

HELPING YOURSELF .

At the end of the day, it's your own illness. And most definitely, your own body. I found it was really important to listen to it.

It's very tempting to hand over responsibility for yourself to others when you're ill. Doctors, nurses, specialists, societies, anyone really, that you feel might know more about your illness than you do.

Obviously, all these people have an important role to play, but in the end it's YOU that has the most impact on how you feel and how you progress. YOU can help to mend yourself. Nobody knows you as well as you do. Listen to your body — it may only whisper to start with — but you'll start to hear it more and more. Some people call it intuition, others instinct, and others, simply a 'feeling'.

Whatever your symptoms are, it's worth noticing when they happen. Start simply because it doesn't have to be complicated, nor does it need specialised knowledge. Just concentrate on one thing at a time and relax!

However, be warned, it might take a long time. I've been trying to work out what's going on for seven years! You might be better at it than me! Also factors seem to change but that's OK, you'll deal with it.

For example, my right arm was very sensitive. Apart from the permanent pins and needles, sometimes it really hurt deep inside. Sometimes it felt absurdly cold too. I didn't relate the two to begin with but I began to realise there was a link. I learnt to keep my arm covered and warm, whether I was cold or not. Keeping my arm/hand cosseted in this way reduced the sensory signals — less pain, less pins and needles. But wearing a jumper/fleece etc made me too hot and this wasn't any good either. So, once I sussed it, I was to be found with one arm in and one arm out, most of the time. Poor kids, they got incredibly embarrassed walking alongside me down the High Street! Who was this hobo shuffling alongside them in a lop-sided fashion?

A similar example was when my shoulders hurt. This used to happen on and off, over a few months. On the basis that the 'bleeding obvious' might work, I stopped wearing a bra. Blow me down, my shoulders stopped hurting. It was as though the pressure from the straps of the bra on the tops of my shoulders had been spreading out across all the top of my back. It was as though once the straps had turned the nerve receptors on, they stayed on and others joined the party, resulting in some unpleasant sensations.

Diet

My dear old Dad (I haven't mentioned him for a while) used to say, "You are what you eat." I'm not sure what that meant to him, all I remember is he used to talk about "Dr. Dong's" diet, which he swore by to help his arthritis. The mind boggles.

Only you can work out what food suits, or doesn't suit you. I decided that if I couldn't move around much, I should be more careful about what I eat, otherwise I'd end up like a balloon. There are, of course, many diets. They seem to come and go, almost like fashion accessories. The only thing that seems to ring true is that different diets work for different people.

Here's my list. It's just based on my impressions and experiences, some of which are quite old now. In the end, I guess the really useful diets were the ones that taught me something about eating that I could adopt in my everyday life from then on.

- **Weight Watchers** – this helped me a lot because it increased my awareness of the calories contained in many foods. It got me into the habit of counting them. It also featured low fat and processed foods, which as it turned out later I learnt to avoid.
- **Fibre Diet** – this also featured low fat, but, importantly, high fibre. My husband and I used to make up packs and packs of weekly allowances of fibre filler. It looked like hamster food.
- **Slim Fast/Cambridge Diet** – I'm not really sure what to make of these two. They were OK, I suppose, for me. However, I didn't learn anything of lasting value from either. They seemed very insular to me.
- **The Zone Diet**[10]. This was used, apparently, for the American Olympic Swimming Team. I guess they were in pretty good shape anyway. However, it's of interest here because it's quite different – it's about eating equal amounts of protein, carbohydrates and fat. It may seem as though it's not relevant to mere mortals – surely the swimming team will use up all the fat? There may be an element of truth in that, but more interestingly, the diet talks of good, as well as bad, fats. This is far more than the saturated and unsaturated distinction.
- **Kinesology**. This has influenced me the most. Very quickly, I was told things that made sense to me. Mainly this was about

[10] From *Enter the Zone* written by Barry Sears

conserving energy – don't give your body and brain more to handle than you need to[11]. Certainly, I found with MS that I had very little energy, so conserving it seemed a good idea. Mainly, the advice was to eat 'real' food. This meant avoiding processed food. So, controversially, no 'low fat' anything. This included having 'full fat' milk. I beamed. I was so happy. Because I loved milk, butter, cream and hated the ubiquitous synthetic taste of ready-made meals. No wonder it influenced me, I loved it! And, who's to say that wasn't right for me?

Why did I love it? It suited me. And I'm not huge. I'm size 12. Well, 14 at the top. Big (ish) chest, you see.

I decided I'd rather eat less of what I 'fancy', but stick to it, than force myself to eat stuff that I didn't like so much. "A little of what you fancy does you good" – what a useful saying! (My Mum again!)

Fortunately, our son also dislikes pre-prepared food and on the whole the kids seem happy to follow our diet. Although, in fairness, they do supplement it with all the usual – chocolate, crisps, biscuits, chocolate, sweets, fizzy drinks, chocolate, etc. Alan also disappears into the Sacred Heart Cabbage Diet every now and then, which although it's quite controlled, involves a lot of cabbage soup and I'm not sure he fancies that much of it. It is at least 'real'.

I have to say, though, that the "if you fancy it, eat it," philosophy has come unstuck for me a few times. I noticed that bread, particularly French sticks, Chinese food, and horror of horrors – GIN and wine, all did nasty things to me.

In the end, I decided that the first two were due to gluten, which seemed to make my left arm very painful and laid me out flat. I have been avoiding gluten for years, especially bread. If I give in and have even a tiny bit, I feel bloated, heavy and even slower than usual. However, I have to confess to eating pasta – the gluten free pasta that I tried was disgusting – it all stuck together and tasted like cardboard. I can live with the after-effects of 'straight' pasta!

The alcohol was more of a puzzle. I could drink it, but only in tiny quantities. Otherwise, the results were quite dramatic – my arms were OK, but my legs – no. Didn't want to work. And this wasn't about straightforward alcoholic poisoning; my body really had changed since pre-MS days,

[11] This idea ties in with the concept of 'ancestral diet' that Hal Huggins talked about. I mention that in Part 3 under Dental Revision

so the amounts I could drink were now pitiful. Until I learnt that, I used to get upset about the many dirty looks from other people in a restaurant when I went, nay, staggered, to the loo. You could almost hear the 'tuts'. I eventually learnt to take my stick with me to restaurants and use it to go to the toilet – it didn't stop the staggering, but it eliminated the 'tuts'. Anyway, I felt better.

Needless to say, all the above – bread, Chinese, gin and wine – were real favourites of mine. But I had to accept that, while my mind loved them, my body couldn't handle them and told me so very quickly in no uncertain terms.

I had a blood test done for allergies. There appears to be some controversy about the accuracy of these tests, but I found the results interesting. According to this analysis, I was allergic to wheat and yeast. So that explained the bread and wine. I was also allergic to pears and figs. This was more puzzling. I'd never noticed anything about pears, although I suppose I didn't eat them enough to notice any patterns. And figs – I've never eaten one in my life! Maybe that's why. Didn't fancy them!

Sometimes you can find substitutes for things that cause you problems. One of my favourites was fizzy water and grape juice instead of wine, or the *Aqua Libra* product. It was important to me to keep the ritual surrounding the item being substituted – for example; I drank the wine substitute from a really nice wineglass and kept the product in an aesthetically pleasing bottle, on the table. Straightforward and simple maybe, but it really made a difference to me.

Regardless of what I was eating and/or drinking, where and from whatever receptacle, I decided that eating late made the night that followed more restless, with less sleep. So I try to eat by 7pm most of the time.

Drinking

Surprisingly, perhaps, I'm thinking of water here. Feeling shitty? Have a drink of water **before** you feel thirsty. I'm told that your body has to be dehydrated to some extent in order to make you feel thirsty – so don't wait to feel thirsty.

I used to fill up a litre bottle with water every day (they say you're supposed to drink 2 litres a day – I couldn't manage that, but I did what I could) and take it with me everywhere, which really meant round the house! When I went out, I had a smaller bottle of water with me all the time, even if I was just popping out for half an hour. I kept it in the car and sometimes I strapped it to my wheelchair.

I do all this less now, it doesn't seem so important any more, but the real reason may be that I now suffer a lot from needing to urinate in an increasingly urgent way.

The water I drank (and still do) is filtered water. It's one of the few things I'm adamant about. Tap water tastes disgusting to me now and I can tell if someone has made a cup of tea with water straight out of the tap. (It's not just my taste buds; I can see a dark skin floating on the top of it.)

While we're on drinking, a few thoughts about the grown-up version. Wine, I'm OK with, in moderation! I had an interesting experience with champagne, although I suspect it was the amount that did it – I couldn't walk, you see! Fortunately, I was at home, so when I needed to go to the loo, my husband and son took one armpit each and dragged me there!

But spirits – forget them! I know that even a small amount will 'do for me!' The owner of a local restaurant that I go to a lot offered me a drink. He'd offered before and I'd always turned it down. However, for some reason I decided this was getting churlish of me. So, for once, I agreed. I thought about it for a while, and then decided that a small, and I mean small, port would be lovely. I enjoyed my port, drank it quite quickly and was delighted that it was not having an effect. Then I got the urge to go to the loo and asked my companion for help. (Someone to lean on; get my balance. Perfectly normal for me.) Well, what a trial! I simply could not move my legs – I screamed at them inside my head, but they may as well have belonged to someone else – they took no notice at all. Waiters were offering to help and I was getting more and more desperate to go! Anyway, it wasn't far and I managed to get there – just about. But, no more port.

Exercise

I believe that exercise is really important. The difficulty is that 'exercise', i.e. the reasons for it and the resultant benefits, are not the same if you have MS, as they are if you haven't. With MS I was practising getting neural messages through, not strengthening muscles.

So, for me, the whole principle was not about fitness, health, beauty and keeping in shape. Of course, my stomach might disagree with that.

Another monumental event that affected me was totally unplanned. Basically, I tripped over a rug in my own hallway, messing up my knee. It had to be the left one – the same side that is worse affected by MS. Still, look on the bright side, at least I didn't rip my ligaments on the other leg – then I'd have had problems with both legs!

I had keyhole surgery on my messed up knee, but, to be honest, it didn't get better. Maybe it would have been worse without the surgery, but I think I expected too much. I think the term 'key-hole', plus the lack of a big scar made me feel that less had happened to me than actually had inside. Four years on and I still couldn't walk right. I know I should exercise my leg more, so that my knee has some muscles to hold onto. But I hate exercise – it's *so* boring and yes, I know I should – but…

Back to the learning to walk exercises …

Peace and Quiet

I guess you don't have to have MS to like a bit of this! The ability to be in a quiet and peaceful place varies for all of us, I'm sure. I just know that for me, I have to work at it.

One of my main problems is the T.V. – my husband and kids walk into a room, turn the telly on and leave it on, even if they're leaving the room. We, like most UK households, have more than one telly – start to get the picture? (Sorry, another pun!)

My brain can be truly messed up with music – from stereos, radios or the computer. Don't get me wrong, I love music but not opera. Sorry, but I don't. I have tried. My family plays some good stuff but somehow it addles my brain. I find it difficult to process – it almost hurts. Especially if I can hear more than one source of music or sound at once. (Try sitting at the bottom of our stairs – it'll make your brain boggle – MS or not.)

Also, I have big problems with talk radio – I just can't think of anything else while I'm trying to comprehend the insistent whittering.

And, love them as I do, the dogs' barking drives me (and our neighbours) crazy. Still, guarding the place is Maggie, the Alsatian's job, while the West Highland white terrier, Max, joins in to show willing and because she told him to.

I thought about showing you pictures of the animals, but there was only one that I thought summed up the remarkably easy truce and tolerance that they all seem to share:

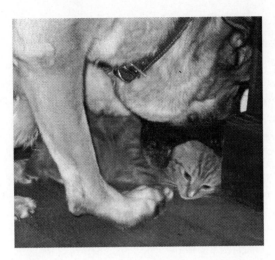

I've tried to explain to my family how the noises and movement can almost physically hurt me. I certainly find it even more difficult to walk if any of the above are distracting me. It's almost as though I only have limited brain space available – use some up processing sound and there's less available for other things – like balancing.

It's a real pain and I wish it didn't matter – but it does.

Temperature Control

I'm told that this is a typical problem for people with MS, although I'm not sure why.

Never mind, it certainly is odd. Why, for example, in the middle of winter am I the only one in the High Street with no overcoat on? It's because my body isn't able to keep my temperature down. This is important because parts of me, particularly my legs and balance, don't work when I'm too hot.

Another point: I learnt that your temperature goes up by one degree (centigrade, I think) when you eat a meal. That might explain why it can be REALLY HARD to get upstairs, even with help, directly after supper. Some people have mentioned that getting a stair-lift (like the one that Thora Hird helps advertise) would help. Undoubtedly it would. However, the exercise of going up the stairs feels important to me, and I'm loath to give it up. I feel too young for that! If I wait for a couple of hours[12] and really cool down, then getting upstairs is much easier.

As another way of controlling temperature, I'd like to say "blankets". I

---

[12] Watch some TV or a good film – something to take my mind off going to bed, lying down and finishing the day.

know that I forgot about blankets in this age of duvets but they really have helped me control my temperature at night. This isn't exactly rocket science either, but having stayed at a hotel with blankets on the bed, I realised that was much better for me. I could easily change the temperature of the bed by a few degrees by shedding or adding a blanket rather than freeze or burn with a duvet[13], which could only be off or on.

So, not only is it a problem being too hot, but being too cold isn't tolerable either. It's as though activating the nerves carrying the 'too cold' messages trigger off nerves which deal with pain. That's why I can be seen to sport a woolly scarf around my left knee every night, even in the summer. My feet, too, can be painfully cold; hence the hot water bottle every night, regardless of the season.

Generally, it seems my body is bad at generating its own heat and that's why I've come to rely on external sources of heat such as the scarf or hot water bottles. I've tried an electric blanket but that was disastrous: heat all over, which made some bits of me too hot!

I've referred to temperature control problems in other sections as well as here, but I also wanted to mention the twenty-minute rule. I'm reminded that on last year's holiday to Northern Cyprus, where the temperature was in the 40's, instinctively I was uncomfortable lying in the sun for more than 20 minutes. I didn't have a watch on but it seemed that my body clock was pretty accurate. I only lay out in the sun once, at most twice, a day. I'm really sorry if you find tanning hard, but this regime resulted in a great tan.

Looking back, I realise that at the time I was on holiday I hadn't yet experienced the 20-minute rule. It just felt right to me. Later on the rule re-emerged since it was proposed by both the ex-dentist and physicist that I talk about in Part Three.

Sleep

Word out seems to be that sleep is when we heal. If, with MS, it's true that your immune system is attacking your myelin sheath[14], then sleep seems more important than ever.

Like stress, I suspect that we only understand half of it, at best.

I know my sister didn't sleep at all well for years. She used to try and sleep through the night, but kept waking at about two in the morning. Then she would take half a 'Tamazepan' in order to sleep for some of the

---

[13] And I've tried a few different togs, I can tell you!

[14] I have come across some people who have their doubts about this. I'm not sure either. Just on logical grounds – how can "remission" (as in remitting/recurring MS) occur if the sheath has been so badly damaged?

rest of the night. She only took half because she was scared they were addictive.

Having been through the addictive thing with Zopiclone, I can understand what she was worried about. However, good sleep is paramount and there are other ways of promoting it, like:

- having a bath (although for me, there came a point when getting in and out was too much hard work and it made me too hot!)
- the smell of lavender (maybe as oil sprinkled on your pillow or just in a bowl by your bed).
- reading (sometimes something boring works).
- a mug of warm milk (my Dad swore by this!)

or, most effective of all for me, a non-addictive sleeping pill[15].

[15] Although the effect would wear off after about 3 nights. So, 2/3 nights off, then back on again, off, on etc., seems to work.

ALTERNATIVE THERAPIES

I've tried all kinds of therapies and met some stunning practitioners while doing so.

Physiotherapy

Having been to quite a few physiotherapists, it's quite clear that if you have MS (and maybe other similar conditions) then you need to go to a **Neurological Physiotherapist.** Even if a Physio understands the problems of fatigue that people with MS encounter, it's unlikely that you will get the right exercises to help the condition, unless the physio is trained as a neurological physiotherapist.

I remember the first lady physio I had with great affection and respect. She was a neuro physio and appeared to understand my problems and how to try and fix them. She dissected walking down to a fine art and my exercises were designed to replicate the various elements of walking. We met way back in 1998, and I've lost touch with her for some years now. However, I've still got a few of her exercises. Here's a flavour of them (but I take no responsibility for them if you try them...)

1. Pelvic Wiggle
Move hips side to side – each side x6
Stay up tall, shoulders still.

2. Standing Balance
Stand in front of work surface/table
Hands in crab (– in case lose balance – hands nails down, palm towards table – hand looks like a crab)
Stand on alternate legs for balance
Repeat twice each leg.

3. One Leg Shorter than the other
Watch hip in front of mirror. Hold on.
Swap legs.

4. Tip toes
Pull in stomach and bum.

Up and down on tip toes – both legs at once.
Imagine crown of head being pulled straight up.

I also remember going to the National Hospital for Neurological Diseases (where I was first diagnosed) in 2002. It was really exciting to meet a physio who knew what he was doing in relation to MS. I can't stress enough how vastly different this type of therapist is to a 'physio' as we would usually imagine them. They appear to work on a different level, focusing on the nervous system, not on muscles. So they concentrate on the conduction of signals in the body in terms of sensation, co-ordination and feedback.

For example, he quickly worked out that while my left leg wasn't so well co-ordinated (which I had already been told) my right leg (which I'd always thought of as the 'normal' one) had problems feeding back to me where it was in space. I don't mean that it was off circling the planet but more that it could misjudge its position in relation to the rest of me by one or more inches. This was certainly contributing to my balance problems.

And my exercising concentrated on stabilising my pelvis and using my stomach muscles to move around – sit down, stand up, moving from side to side and walking. It's amazing how much I tried to move in these ways by using my shoulders! Again, here's a taster. But same provisos – beware!

Do a little, 5 minutes, often. (Avoid fatigue.)

1. Sit and alternate:
Sink – slouch with pelvis – shoulders relaxed, palms up
Rise – straighten back from pelvis – shoulders relaxed, palms up

2. Lift each leg, in turn, while sunk

Balance exercises.
REMEMBER – DO EVERYTHING SLOWLY

3. Standing by firm surface, feet together, facing surface, bottom and tum pulled in,
    a) raise alternative arms over head X10.
    b) close eyes – 1 minute.

4. Standing sideways onto surface, one foot in front of the other, trying to maintain balance for a minute. Swap feet and repeat.

5. Standing by bottom stair, holding on to rail, one foot on step, bend knee of lower leg you're standing on, so that its knee goes forward over toes. X 10.
Swap legs and repeat.

You can see how different they are to 'ordinary' (i.e. non-neurological MS) physio exercises. When my walking gets awful, I go back to them. They appear to help.

Recently, I've met a physio at the Royal Free who understands MS beyond the fatigue issue. Not surprisingly she's a member of the neurology team and it does make a big difference. The exercises she gave me are fairly basic and are about learning to use new nerve pathways and the feedback sensations that occur when you do. Hopefully, these grow to become automatic.

I can't stress sufficiently that we don't have enough neuro physios in the U.K. – either privately or on the NHS. I was lucky in that I lived in North London, which meant it was relatively easy to find them, but many people don't have such easy access. My sister didn't. Let's start a campaign and demand more of them, dotted all over the U.K.

Stomach exercises / Swimming

I used to try and do stomach exercises on the floor. I own up, I found them very boring and I couldn't do very many of them. So when our very playful and big Alsatian decided to join in, I was really glad! All exercise just had to stop!

Now I do more swimming. Well, I don't actually swim – I was banned from doing breaststroke because of my knee ligaments (which I told you about earlier) and while a dear friend is trying to teach me front crawl – it's slow. I don't really like putting my head in the water, so it would be!

But being in the water is fabulous. No need to balance. I get a tremendous feeling of freedom, just floating about or even just walking from side to side down the shallow end. Doesn't hurt when you fall over, you see.

If you could go swimming without getting wet, it would be perfect! Roll on zero gravity tanks.

Massage

I love a massage. Swedish massage is the one for me. Fairly deep, into the tissues, but not brutal. And pummelling is definitely out for me. I once went through an experience where the 'masseuse' stood on me – I can't remember what type of massage that was called, but it wasn't for me. My friend tried it and loved it! We're all different, I guess!

I've been lucky enough to have a couple of friends who have been properly trained and do a great massage. I was a 'body' for one of them for her exam. At the moment, the other one comes round to my house about once a week to give me a massage at a reduced 'friend' rate. Jammy bugger me, long may it continue! I'm sure, though, if I'd gone round to the local college where they teach massage, I could have met someone who had recently qualified or was due to qualify soon, and let them practise on me!

On a more serious note, I feel quite energised after a massage. It may in part be due to the fact that I'm lying down flat for an hour, but I think the feedback of the sensations from all over my body wakes me up. I'm told that most 'normal' people feel sleepy after a massage, but not me!

I'm also told that massage helps keep your muscles toned. I must say no one has ever told me that my leg muscles are weak, so maybe it's the massage that has helped keep them strong. It beats exercise, I know that!

Cranial Osteopathy

I've been going to a cranial osteopath, a lovely man called Gez, for almost two decades now. I find it fascinating.

I was first introduced to cranial osteopathy when I was pregnant with Tom. I remember it very clearly: it was a meeting of the 'bump club' on a cold winter's day with a lot of snow on the ground. Not many of us got to the gathering, so the cranial osteopath who was running the session decided to demonstrate using each of us in turn. One by one he got the women to lie on their back on the floor and he cradled their head in his hands. He talked about past traumas that had happened to people, the effect that this may still have and any other ailments that were troubling them. He didn't get it all right, but there were quite a few things that he mentioned from people's pasts, plus present-day things that were troubling them, that none of us knew about.

It was fairly impressive. My MS wasn't noticeable then and I was delighted that he didn't mention it when it came to my turn. I nearly avoided my turn altogether, but he spied me hiding in the corner!

Cranial Osteopathy is based on the undeniable principle that every part of us is connected together. It centres on a rhythm that the practitioner can feel in the head where the part of your skull that is called the fontanel in babies has not quite fused together. So, in the same way as we all have a breathing rhythm and a heart beat, there's also a cranial rhythm. Since the body is all connected, the rhythm in the skull apparently informs about how the rest of the body is. There are three aspects to this rhythm – the rate, the balance and the stability. There is also a belief that body tissues have a 'memory.' For example muscles etc. can remember how it felt to be injured and may still be compensating for this, even if the original injury was years ago. So part of the therapy can be getting the tissues to let go of these memories. It doesn't have to involve physical manipulation. The therapist, by giving help in the form of some kind of energy, can encourage the patient to heal him or herself.

I've known these principles apply to purely psychological events that have happened in the past too. For example, there was someone who I increasingly felt uncomfortable with, to the extent that fear began to take over. During a C.O. session, I remembered that this person reminded me of a relative who touched me sexually when I was eight. Just remembering seemed to release the tension, or whatever it was, and my disquiet about this person evaporated.

Over the years, I've been to see Gez many times and given other people the contact too. He's always helped people with a whole multitude of problems – from being in a coma to backache. I've watched him treat babies too – once the 'bump club' had produced its many and various offspring. Both Tom and Alice have been to see him and reaped benefits from doing so.

The remaining question is – can cranial osteopathy help my MS? It can certainly help calm me down, not just emotionally, but also physically, since it seems to physically stop my nerves from 'buzzing'. I have come out of some sessions being able to walk better than I could when I first arrived. But there's a limit to what I can expect from any one thing, I think. The cranial osteopath said he started off believing there was nothing he could do for MS, but finally thinks it may be possible to help at least.

Schneider Self-Healing

A friend first drew my attention to Meir Schneider and his approach to self-healing and then I discovered that a lady who had been trained in this technique/philosophy lived nearby. I just had to go and see her.

I visited her several times and enjoyed every consultation. Each time lasted 1-2 hours and included a discussion of my condition[17], some massage and some movements/exercises.

To be honest, I didn't do this technique justice. I liked and identified with the ideas involved such as the body's ability to heal itself, the importance of taking control/responsibility for your own body/illness and trying to understand and listen to what your body tells you. The problem was that I was not disciplined enough to devote an hour or so per day to doing the required movements/exercises.

More fool me, you might say. I bought the book[18] with every good intention. I read some of it and intend to read more – I'm waiting to find the time and energy to do so[19].

Clairvoyant Healer

This person was also fascinating since she was unlike anyone I'd met before. After two sessions, she decided she couldn't help me because my energy levels were too low. However, she did tell me that my aura indicated that I was a healer. "Maybe I could start with myself," I thought.

She also said that creativity was very important to me. This was of most interest to me since it intuitively felt right. I was already painting, both ceramics and watercolour, and had done a little bit of writing. Her comments spurred me on to do more of these things, and I do feel better (relatively) when I do.

Spiritual Healer

This was the weirdest of all. The lady, who I saw about ten times, was dressed in white, like a nurse you see on American TV programmes. She was lovely, short and very approachable. At the time that I saw her both my parents had died, although my sister was still alive.

I spent our sessions lying on the therapy table with my eyes shut, while she stayed mainly around my head. She said nothing and neither did I. Unless I wanted to.

During my second session with her, I was suddenly aware of a ball of fire, about the size of a football, floating beside me. It didn't burn; it was just a bundle of energy. I found myself talking to my Mum, telling her that I always thought she was closer to my sister than to me.

I also apologised for being in a bad mood the last time we met before

---

[17] More whittering.
[18] *The Handbook of Self-Healing* by Meir Schneider and Maureen Larkin
[19] Feeble excuse

she died. This was important to me since she died very suddenly. She was killed by a lorry that caught the side of the bus just where she was sitting. Ironically, she had changed places with her sister moments before the accident. This was because her sister was deaf in one ear and couldn't hear my mum speaking.

Obviously we only found this out from her sister Connie who did survive, although her shoulder and arm were hurt. I don't know if my Auntie Connie felt bad about changing places. It made sense to me that Mum, who had already lost her husband (and hated it) should die rather than Connie, whose husband was still alive at the time. Also, I liked to think that my Dad 'knew' how miserable my Mum was and sort of 'welcomed her up to join him'.

Mum died 15 months after my Dad died. At least she met Alice, albeit for just over a year. Tom was nearly five when she died.

The funeral was held 'up North', Middlesborough, to be precise. I don't remember very much about it. Except that it was unreal. Did the coffin that they wheeled in and then rollered off to the incinerator after the service, really contain my Mum?

Back to the Healer. Given the circumstances, it makes sense that I needed to 'address' my Mum. So the 'ball of fire', which, just to clarify, I felt more than saw[20], represented her. She always had a lot of energy – my Dad was always saying, "Sit down, Jane". Just watching her wore the rest of us out. Talking to her at the Healer's made me feel as though I'd made 'peace' with her.

This aspect about my mum was the most important thing that emerged from my spiritual healer sessions. They stopped because the lady didn't approve of the steroid treatment I was about to have and decided she could not help me any more.

---

[20]That would have terrified me.

FIGHTING FATIGUE –
MAKING LIFE MORE TOLERABLE

As well as the intense frustration of having limbs and other things not working, there has been the annoyance of fatigue. This isn't like normal fatigue, it's not that you feel tired, it's that you just CAN'T do anything, let alone stay upright or even sit down. I think it's called 'chronic' fatigue.

Four things have helped me here – lying down, darkness, quiet and drinking water. All four together seem to be necessary to 'rest'. Taking a drug called Amantadine has also helped reduce the fatigue.

I think a good rest boils down to being comfortable. Until I began to understand my body better, I felt like the leading lady in the 'Princess and the Pea.' I don't know what someone had placed below whatever I was lying on, but I could feel every tiny bump and irregularity. You'd think it would be easy, but it took me ages to work it all out and get into a routine so that it was all 'comfy' fairly automatically whenever it was 'rest' time. Now I'm almost fanatical about some things, so I expect I'm a real pain to live with at times.

Lying Down

For me, this had to be lying down absolutely flat. It's as though my body benefits from having less work to do; inactivity, plus no balancing and less pumping of blood against gravity. I've also found that 20 minutes is the magic time that I need to lie down for; 15 or so minutes is not enough and 25-30 minutes has no incremental benefits.

Importantly, I don't need to sleep during this time. Sometimes I do, for whatever time I need, and I guess then sleep is beneficial, but the lying down works without the sleep too.

Darkness

An aversion to light has been with me since 1998. Certainly light sources – like an electric light or a bright window – cause me problems. The light seems to sear into my brain and make it boggle.

The answer to this has always been fairly simple: a really comfortable blindfold. I take my blindfold away with me everywhere. Or, failing that, I use the corner of a pillow or cushion.

Unfortunately, this doesn't work when I'm trying to watch the telly. The problem is when the TV is the light source in an otherwise darkened room[21], so another light has to be on.[22] Our daughter, Alice, has a similar problem – she feels like the movement on the TV in a dark room might set off her migraine.

Drinking Water

I know I've mentioned water already, but just a couple of big gulps before you lie down seem to help enormously.

Amantadine

I originally found information about this on the U.S. Multiple Sclerosis web site. Apparently it's man-made dopamine; we all use this naturally as a catalyst for generating impulses along our nerves. Since those with MS appear not to be very good at communicating along their nerve cells, help of this kind made sense to me.

I had to ask for it, though. I think there's some mixed feelings about it amongst the medical profession.

Incidentally, the drug also has anti-viral properties – that would explain why in the winter everyone in our household gets colds and coughs, except for me! Well, won one at least!

When I first got the drug, I wasn't sure whether to take one or two a day. I was afraid that I wouldn't be able to sleep if I took two. So, typical of me, I kept a diary in the hope that I could see a pattern and work it out. The diary begins with my concern about a sleeping tablet that I'd been on for a long time. I've left it in because I think sleep can be a problem for people – it certainly was for my sister, as well as for myself.

Friday 22nd March 2002

I'm writing this at 3 o'clock in the morning – something I haven't done since I was working, about 4 years ago.

Normally, I'd talk to my counsellor – but I haven't seen her for a while and she would, quite rightly, kill me if I phoned her now!

I'm confused about what's going on with me, the effect of some new (for me) drugs, and what I should do now.

---

[21] Unless we're watching a scene in a graveyard at night or a dark basement. So, Dracula movies are OK, as was "Silence of the Lambs," especially at the end.
[22] We can't have the fish-tank lights on either though – in the dark, it's too distracting! Apart from the fact that I swear I saw them all lined up at one end of the tank watching a wild-life programme, it's right next door to the telly and it's distracting!

I'll set out what's been happening, or at least my view of it:

Sept 2001 – from thinking I might actually be able to get better, I'm now starting to feel worse! I'm finding that I sleep worse with the stronger dose (7.5 mg) of Zopiclone[23], and also with the weaker one (3.75 mg). The high dose makes me very drowsy in the morning; with the low dose I wake up 3 - 4 times a night. I do this to go to the loo, and maybe one time every night I'll stay awake for an hour or so. But I never before got up at 3 in the morning to type!

After about a year on these tablets, I went to see my GP – who very brightly suggested I take half of the high and half of the low every night. So my dose was 5.625 mg (3.75 + 1.875) every night. Not that my husband's cutting was that accurate, but roughly it was about right. The halves tasted disgusting, so I took them buried in honey (it has to be Greek!) and brushed my teeth afterwards every night. This all worked a treat. I wasn't drowsy in the morning and I only woke up 1 - 2 times a night, and didn't stay awake for an hour or so a night so often.

I stayed like this for about four months – it got me through Christmas. (Not easy at the best of times!)

However, just after Christmas I noticed how slow and fatigued I'd become and how much more I slept during the day. This was only for about an hour but while before I'd just rested horizontally for 20-30 minutes, these rest/sleeps were longer.

Some while later, my disquiet about the increased fatigue resurfaced. It occurred to me that maybe the Zopiclone was making me more useless during the day. I also harboured the feeling that I ought to ditch it if I could. After all, I'd been on it nearly two years. So, following my success with half-and-half, amounting to around 5 mg, I decided to take the low tablet every night. I was happily on 3.75 mg for a couple of weeks. And then I went down to half a low one, 1.875-ish mg. But the fatigue was still there, if anything, getting a bit worse. What was strange was that my sleep was, if anything, getting better the less Zopiclone I took. During my fortnight of the lowest dose I actually slept all the way through the night a couple of times.

During my disquiet, one Saturday morning I woke up and felt so fed up with the fatigue I was experiencing, that I looked up

[23] A strong, highly addictive sedative. It was first prescribed for me immediately after my first oral dose of steroids, because I had hardly slept for a month. Horrible. What a great way to start the new millennium!

"Multiple Sclerosis" on the Internet. Ping, I went straight into the North American Multiple Sclerosis page. After wandering about for a short time I came across a list of symptoms and highlighted Fatigue. There I found a description of how I'd been feeling. Well, - ish. It was close and made the distinction between 'ordinary' fatigue and MS 'fatigue', which is very hard for an outsider to understand. My kids have great difficulty with it – it's way outside their realm of experience. They say, "but I'm tired too, I've been at school all day." (Which I make worse by mentally adding – unlike you, mother, who's been sitting at home all day, with nothing that you have to do!)

Also on this web site was a drug, Amantidine, which they said had helped some patients with 'MS fatigue'. I felt I needed to try this.

In late February I went to see my consultant. He suggested I took a different sleeping tablet, so I could come off the Zopiclone. Once I had built this up, across 4 weeks, I could take Amantidine. I wanted to come off Zopiclone anyway and I nearly had, so I was happy with this plan.

I spent the next week waiting for an appointment with my GP who needed to prescribe the drugs and used the time to finish off my anti-Zopiclone plan that I reduced to 0 mg for the week. I slept fine – woke up 1 - 2 times a night for a pee and then straight back to sleep again.

I got the alternative sleeping tablet (Amitriptyline) from my doctor, and expressed my confusion and doubt about going onto another sleeping tablet, especially since I'd just got off Zopiclone. She suggested I phone the consultant and see what he thought.

I tried one new sleeping tablet (apparently an anti-depressive, although he didn't think I was depressed, but it would help me sleep). I woke up 3 times in the night and took about an hour to go back to sleep again. I also felt very groggy in the morning.

This didn't feel like an advance so I didn't take any more, and spent the rest of the week without Zopiclone as well.

I phoned the consultant, who was very helpful. He explained that the other sleeping tablet was not addictive since it was not a derivative of valium, like Zopiclone was. Also he thought that if I got a decent night's sleep with Amitriptyline then my fatigue might go away. He also said he didn't feel strongly about the plan and I could just go to the Amantidine anti-fatigue pill tomorrow if I wanted to.

So I think I want to go straight to the anti-fatigue drug. The consultant called it a "Wake-up" drug but on the Internet it said no one understands how MS fatigue works, but that Amantidine <u>does</u> work for some people. So let's hope that Amantidine reduces my fatigue without making me buzz like the steroids did in 1999.

After all that's how I got onto Zopiclone in the first place.

But let's be more positive – Amantidine is something else!

Monday 25th March 2002

Much to my delight and relief my GP called me on Friday, and wrote a prescription for Amantidine, which I picked up that afternoon.

I scheduled out what I took, the effect and what happened. I won't bore you with the detail; it's deadly dull. Suffice it to say I went on to note:

It's only a few days but I do feel better – it's as though a chemical is back in my body that hasn't been there for 4 years. A chemical I need to access my energy resources in a positive way. Maybe a catalyst? I haven't put weight on much these past four years, although I have eaten less, probably. My stomach sags like an ageing man's paunch, but that's the only place (I think!)

Somehow the MS stopped me from using my energy. It's supposed to eat away at your myelin sheath that covers your nerves. This must be a protein. Maybe it also attacks other protein molecules in your body – one could be a catalyst.

Whatever, I feel much better. I'm not using my stick and I feel I can face the world again. Plans that were daunting now seem possible:

- exercises from neurological physiotherapist.
- exercise ball especially for stomach – at least I feel like pumping it up now[24].
- building project at home not so daunting – although I still need help.
- maybe, eventually, I'll take the final two years of my

---

[24] The ball, not my stomach! Although I think my stomach's already been blown up – some gremlin in the night!

counselling training. So at least I'm qualified, and so could do it …

And my biggest problem is going to be not to overdo it. Guilt drives me on, so I need to check with whoever I'm feeling guilty about to see if I'm making them feel bad, or whether the problem is only mine.

Enthusiasm and impatience are culprits too.

I need to keep my calm aura about me and not forget what I've learnt about myself. I'm sure I'll continue to do the learning at least.

How much are we constrained by assumptions?

- The concept that a wake-up drug is the opposite of a go-to-sleep drug?
- That the more you do, the more tired you'll get and the more you'll sleep?

Fatigue is not the same as tiredness. It's something else - it exists outside the dimension of tiredness.

Tiredness:

Wake up – get up – activity all day – get tired – go to sleep.

Fatigue:

Wake up – get up – worn out – got no energy – <u>nothing</u> is easy – lie down for a while – do what you can (not much) – lie down again – go to sleep? Or maybe not, because sleep won't come. Remember that fatigue is not the same as tiredness.

Although the two tablets a day don't seem to have woken me up. (Why am I typing this at 10 p.m. then?) It may be that getting up at 9 and doing more, resting only for 20 minutes all day, actually results in wanting to sleep just as much as taking one tablet a day.

But there are other factors which dictate whether we sleep or not. I'm typing this at 2.28 am on Thursday morning (28th) after lying awake for an hour and a half. This is after taking one tablet, not two like before. I think I'm awake because I'm excited, whereas before I was unhappy and on edge. So agitation will disturb my sleep, whether it's positive or negative, although the former is clearly more pleasant and less frustrating while you're lying awake.

Anyway, seeing a new neurological physiotherapist is what has got me excited and is keeping me awake.

I kept the diary for several weeks and true to scientific form, concluded:

- I'm not sure there is a pattern.
- There's more to sleep than the drugs! Lots to think about, being excited. Also, cats, dogs and children.
- Having only one tablet doesn't mean I get a good night's sleep – I do that with 2 or 1.

I haven't done my diary now for a fortnight, and I'm left thinking that the main pattern is all about consistency – that I need to keep the same daily dose – swapping around just seems to confuse my body. Two a day seems right too, otherwise late afternoon/evening is difficult and that's bad if I'm driving then. So I think I'll settle down to 2 a day.

It's worth remembering too that many things that affect me are normal for 'normal' people. Like having a cold, or a period – they'll pull me down like anyone else. It's just that my starting point is lower. Also, if they both start together then it's very yucky!

POSITIVE THINKING

Just recently I kept getting stuck on the floor after I'd fallen over. I'm told my balance is shot, so I think it's that, not because my legs have 'gone!'.

But being stuck like that really turns the tears on. I feel so helpless, so useless and so sorry for myself; not to mention how unfair life is – why me?

But that approach can't last. Where would it get me?

So, when I get stuck, I have to concentrate on the things that I **can** still do. "Count your blessings", as my dear old Mum used to say.

So with that spirit in mind, I've included my thoughts on being on holiday, back in 2001.

Going on Holiday

VERY GOOD, MUM! (My son's comment about what I've written – I'm proud of it, so I kept it in!)

These are my thoughts upon arriving* in Greece:

Mainly that I'm delighted to get here – there were minimal delays – an hour's wait on the tarmac for flight clearance – that was OK. But most importantly, **I'm chuffed to be here.**

the 'assistance' route helped hugely again – once I swallowed my pride and let myself become someone who is 'assisted', it worked a treat. I don't know if it's sacrilege to say it but I even have fun in a wheelchair, or, in airports, on the electric carts that go "beep, beep". The world changes dramatically – in terms of the physical view you have and the kindness people show when they realise there is a person who talks and, importantly, laughs and jokes.

I have lots of thoughts about being in a wheelchair – a couple of pages later.

If you don't go on holiday or away for a change of scene, list out why. When you break down the elements of travelling (abroad or otherwise) that stop you or that worry you, you may think of ways to overcome them, bit by bit.

---

* This was my second holiday in Greece. Well, that's not true. I had numerous holidays on various islands when I was 'normal', and, it has to be said, younger! This is my second post MS Greek holiday.

My list was:

- I can't get too hot. My ability to control my own temperature, particularly downwards, was seriously impaired. To begin with, I thought that all warm/hot climes were off limits to me now. However, I needed to remember the wonders of air-conditioning. America seems to be completely air-conditioned – the homes, the malls, the shops, the cars. Only the outdoors seems to be beyond their control, for now.
- But air-conditioning has reached other places too. Even Greece. This was unthinkable in my backpacking days but it's true! We found it in a beautiful island called Paxos, just south of Corfu. But I bet it's in other places too, just ask. And get assurances it will work relentlessly when you're there.
- I need to lie down at frequent intervals – a long haul flight was too long, especially overnight.
- Holidays changed to short haul destinations – Greece instead of Florida.
- When I went long haul to South Africa, which was an eleven-hour flight, in effect I shortened it by taking sleeping pills – it worked like a dream (if you'll pardon the pun). It turned into a three hour flight
- I can't walk far at all – the hike to the 'departure gate' at all airports can take for 'ever' – the 'beep buggy' can help hugely or a wheelchair. Ask for assistance when you book your tickets and it'll be set up ready for you when you check in.
- For all types of holiday, still ask about a wheelchair or assistance – there may be more available than you think. Or, for the wheelchair, either buy (about £200 – £400) or rent one (about £10 for one day – delivered to and collected from your home).

Having been on holiday now for almost a fortnight some other thoughts occur:

- Since I'm normally without the family most days at home – kids are at school, husband at work – compared to normal, a holiday is a rest for them but work for me. I think this is a problem for me

– I try and keep up with them and do too much. They're very good and understand – it's me that's had trouble seeing it.

- Similarly, as my son pointed out, I need to adjust my rest times. Resting when they're active, doing things that I can't – like Tennis – is better than me doing something, even if it's reading. The home routine, which is based on timings of school runs and cooking tea doesn't work. By adjusting it on holiday I'm more 'with it' when they're around – so in the evening for example, I can play cards until 11 p.m. And much to everyone's surprise, I was quite good. See, MS doesn't necessarily, or irrevocably, melt your brain.

Being in a Wheelchair

It took me a couple of years to get used to the idea of using a wheelchair. I guess that, like a blue disabled badge for a car, a wheelchair strongly signalled to me an inferior being – someone who could not do, **or think**, as much as the 'norm' (whatever that is).

I now try to think of both a blue badge and a wheelchair as tools that help me do things more easily. That's all.

As suggested, when I was talking about a holiday in the previous section, I first used a wheelchair to get round an airport. And, I confess, I enjoyed it!

The next step was to use one of the wheelchairs that were available at Brent Cross Shopping Centre. Despite what my husband might tell you, I'm not a great one for retail therapy but I've had many experiences shopping in a wheelchair at this shopping centre.

To begin with I was very self-conscious in a wheelchair. I felt embarrassed and like I was some kind of freak. On the whole, people got out of the way of the wheelchair – which was very nice since it made it easier to get around.

But if they had to be with me in a lift or in a shop they might shout as though I was deaf or daft. Either that or ignore me because I wasn't in their line of sight – wrong height – or because they didn't know what to say or do.

I have to confess that I was probably guilty of doing the same sort of things when confronted with someone in a wheelchair in my pre-MS days. So, I wasn't cross about it. It just seemed rather sad.

But I quickly realised, just like public speaking (of which I've done a fair amount [25]) that the 'power' lies with the person in the spotlight (wheelchair!).

I also decided to buy my own wheelchair. (I had to ignore the nagging little voice in my head that kept saying, "Ooh, does that mean I REALLY AM DISABLED?") It was a hassle hiring it all the time, so I made enquiries and found one that was fairly new, ex-rental and PURPLE![2]

So I stopped dreading the experience, and started having fun. It wasn't difficult. Smiling at people made a big difference, just as it does if you're perfectly 'able'. Or saying something, anything, to break the ice in a lift or in a queue virtually always got a positive response. On the whole, being in a wheelchair, or even just using a walking stick, prompts some really friendly, funny and helpful reactions from people. Most people are really nice – provided you are too. However, I must reiterate what two ladies, both of whom are permanently in wheelchairs and I now count as friends, said,

"You want to watch that you don't get into that chair too much ...
I did, and that was twenty years ago."

Making Yourself Feel Better (however briefly)

There are times when we all need some help to put it back together again. There are lots of ways that people make themselves feel better – I'm sure you've already got some of your own!

Appreciating the natural beauty of things around you – this sounds rather trite but it works a treat – and it's free! If you just sit and look around you, you can see things which, when appreciated, and really looked at, can make you feel better. A house plant, a photograph, a piece of china – anything that you enjoy looking at. You don't have to go anywhere, just stay put.

Some people enjoy going for a drive in the country for the same reason – looking at trees, scenery, etc.

It's a strong, but simple idea. The Celestine Prophecy[26] talks a lot about the energy that can be derived from appreciating things that you find beautiful.

---

[25] At conferences, on the radio (once!) and the television (four times, although you could only see my feet and hear my voice). The TV broadcast really confused Tom and Ali since it was recorded and we were watching it all together when it came on-air. Alice, who was all of 3 at the time said, "Mummy, that lady (pointing at the TV) has your shoes on... and she sounds like you!" I tried to explain that it was me, but to 3 and 6 year olds it did not compute – how could I be sitting next to them and be over on the telly at the same time?

[26] Unfortunately, only the metal frame was purple – the rest was black.

[27] The Celestine Prophecy written by James Redfield.

Another idea is to help someone else. There's a therapeutic value to feeling needed. Whatever skill you have[28] – listening, talking, writing, numeracy, proof reading, thinking – someone should appreciate your help. Not that it's easy to volunteer – it took me ages to find organisations that would accept me.

Some other people go and do something they know they're going to enjoy to cheer themselves up. You know what that is better than anyone else – reading maybe, gardening, baking, sewing.

My Dad used to go into the garage, swear like a trooper, and strip down, wait for it … the lawnmower engine.

Talking of lawnmowers, I remember one Saturday afternoon when a boyfriend turned up on his motorbike in all his leathers. As he walked up to our front door he stopped, looked at my Dad who was mowing the lawn and sniffed the air. A short exchange took place between the two of them, which apparently tickled them both! You're thinking that this was about a timely release of body gases, aren't you? No, this was about my Dad using racing oil in the lawnmower! Well, it amused them.

I digress. Really, my main point is to take time to do something for your own sake. It can be anything that helps **you**.

It's not up to other people to judge whether an 'interest' that you have is worthwhile or not. Its value to you is all about you, not someone else. Provided it's not illegal of course. Then you probably would need to reconsider its ultimate value to you!

Don't worry about wasting time either. Or about people thinking you're lazy – you might just be imagining this anyway.

Really, I think this idea is very important!

[28] My sister, who couldn't walk, could type – she did the minutes for the local MS branch meetings.

HELP FROM OTHER SOURCES

Living with someone with MS is, I'm sure, difficult sometimes. It must be hard to know what to do and how to help.

Confidence

As well as physical help, I suspect that helping to build and keep up the MS person's confidence can't be over-emphasised. The kind of nice things that we normally say to each other (hopefully!) become even more important to someone whose body has changed, irrevocably, for the worse.

So, telling the MS person that they look good, or have done something well, really helps. Thanking them for some help they've given another person can also be a huge boost. After all, we are all capable of doing something to help – even if it's just making a phone call.

I'm not suggesting that people become patronising but a bit of reassurance that you're still a worthy member of your community, in whatever way, really helps.

Family

I guess the members of your immediate family are the ones that bear the brunt of the consequences of your MS. They have to get used to the fact that not only can you no longer do the things you used to do for them, but also you need them to do things for you that you would never have dreamt of.

For example, I have needed my teenage kids to clean up after I've urinated on the floor – sort out the puddle, get a change of clothes for me and put my soiled clothes in the washing machine. Did any of us expect that? Both Tom and Alice have risen to the challenge of such occurrences brilliantly. Probably better than I have.

Websites

Not surprisingly, the Internet can be a good source of information, some of which might help you. It's where I first came across the drug Amantadine that has helped me a lot over the years. I just typed in "Multiple Sclerosis", and I got into an American site as well as the MS Society in the U.K. Others that I've used by the time of writing are:

Proventus – a charity dedicated to promoting awareness of Aimspro and Caprivax (Goat serums).

Daval International Ltd – who currently make Aimspro.

ThisIsMS – which refers to itself as "Unbiased Multiple Sclerosis Research, News and Community."

Serono – an American company who are developing products for the treatment of autoimmune diseases.

Multiple Sclerosis – The Greatest Medical Mistake. I thought this was going to be a load of waffle, then my eye caught passages about stress and over-active mental activity during sleep. I had always thought that both of these might have contributed to my problems. Other compounding factors are mentioned as well. The jury's out until I've read the book and investigated its claims.

The MS Society

As I mentioned in the earlier Original Diagnosis section, for many years I didn't go anywhere near the MS Society because I knew how suggestible I could be. However, I know my sister valued the Society a lot and 'worked' for her local branch. Many of the members attended her funeral.

Now, twenty years after being diagnosed, I think it's about time that I joined. This is because while writing this book I realised that I shouldn't bury myself away. Plus, I've developed a stronger sense of myself in relation to MS than I had when I first started this book so I feel less susceptible to suggestions.

Undoubtedly, there are things happening 'out there' that I want to know about. For example, at the time of writing there's much excitement about goat serum, known as Aimspro. Plus I have to say that the MS site is one of the best I've seen; it works, it's user-friendly and it seems 'independent'. Indeed it seems to have won an award for Best Charity site, 2004.

But for all my change in attitude to the society, it still puzzles me when they state that 85,000 people in the UK have MS. I've seen this figure expressed as 1 in 700 people. From my perspective, virtually everyone to whom I've mentioned MS, has known at least one person who has it. Since this has involved talking to virtual strangers as well as friends, I thought that 85K seemed low. Either it was, or I lived in some hyper MS location!

Before joining the Society (which makes about twenty years between diagnosis and joining) I did once have lunch with one of their charming officers. This was at their, then, new offices in North London, and I have to say I was very impressed – both by the people and the facilities. I went not long after I gave up work since I decided that I could use my market research skills to create a questionnaire that would better track people diagnosed with MS. How they felt, what their problems were, how they found help and what else would help them more. It wasn't a medical approach but more of a way to increase understanding about the people with the condition and how they were handling it. The lady I had lunch with was very excited about this idea and took my first-shot questionnaire with her.

I heard no more about this and, in fairness, never pursued it either. Maybe it's time to revisit this issue? The problem is, as it was then, how to identify people with MS who are not members of the Society. I wasn't and I'm sure there are others like me.

Groups

I used to 'run' groups in my former life as a qualitative market researcher. I must have spoken to over ten thousand people in groups of about eight, albeit for only an hour and a half, across the many years I did it. I haven't been a 'respondent' in many groups (they wouldn't have me!) but the few I have been in were difficult for me. I had to stop myself talking too much and, more often than not, stop my trained and natural inclination to take over the group. This helps explain my disinclination to attend any 'self-help groups' that I heard or read about.

However, I did finally join the MS Society. Part of the reason that I joined was because I already knew the local lady who headed up the branch – this was none other than Betty, one of the ladies I went to art classes with for three years! I knew she had something to do with the MS Society but we never talked about it, just painted!

I might go and join in a society group but I also offered my services for running groups for them. We'll see if they take me up on that.

I'VE STILL GOT TO LIVE WITH THIS THING

Having a Bad Time

I've just been through the worst of all the times I've had. I hesitate to say "so far" because it implies it'll happen again, or worse.

It began when my friend, who I was going to the theatre with, simply banned me,

"You're so tired. Your speech is slurred."

And just to make sure, because he knows me too well, he said,

"I'm not going."

He knew that I wouldn't go without him.

It's just as well I didn't go since this was going to be the third time of going to the theatre in a week. I didn't plan it that way – the last play was a short run – a week in the Richmond Theatre. I really wanted to go – I'd never been to a play where I knew the author (a lady actually) but it was clearly a silly idea. I gave in and didn't go.

I felt so holy that night – being sensible – doing the 'right' thing, staying in. My husband and my kids were very pleased that I stayed at home that night. I thought, "I'll be all right in the morning".

True to form, I spoke to my computer shortly afterwards. Here's what I said:

> Morning came – Saturday, thank goodness. I could barely move. I had to really force myself out of bed – I wanted to go to the loo enough to make me shift. At least I could move but I shuffled and waddled like a lame duck. It took ages and much bouncing off walls for me to get the short way to the loo.
>
> And here was me, expecting to feel better than I did the day before. Wrong.
>
> My husband cooked lunch and I forced myself to get up and go downstairs to eat it. After lunch, much to my surprise, I flopped over and had to go back to bed again. I stayed there for the rest of the day. "It's all right," I thought. "I'll be better tomorrow."
>
> Sunday. I woke up, thought, "I'll go to the loo," like I normally do.

Like hell I could. My legs did not want to move. They hurt like they had concrete weights attached to them. I wondered what was going on? Surely I'm better by now?

In the end my screaming bladder shifted my reluctant legs.

I sat on the loo, still wondering. I sniffed, started to blubber with self-pity and blew my nose. I slowly got back into bed.

I started to think about my sister and how she had gone through steadily declining periods when she got worse and worse.

Maybe this was the beginning of my decline?

Maybe I was going to die, like she did?

I wept and wept. How could this be? Maybe it would be a sweet release. No, no. How can that be? I'll leave everyone behind. I won't do that. I WON'T.

OK, OK. I'D OVERDONE IT.

But not this badly, surely? I sniffed. I blew my nose.

Calming myself for a moment, I realised that I had been sniffing and blowing for a couple of days. Not often, otherwise even I would have realised. But it suddenly dawned on me that I had been fighting off a cold for a while. Then I noticed that the glands at the sides of my neck hurt. Maybe it was all this crying? Maybe it was part of the 'cold'?

OK, OK. I'D OVERDONE IT. AND I'D BEEN FIGHTING OFF AN INFECTION.

Last year my GP had advised me to have a flu jab before winter because the immune system doesn't work so well with MS. I had declined, mainly because I didn't want to actively introduce any more to fight. I also remember my Dad complaining about the 'flu that he swears he got from the 'flu jabs he had been given. He was a wonderful 'doubter' of medical men[29] – that's probably where I get a lot of my "I'll do it my way" attitude from.

In the light of this background of defiance and self-reliance, I have been delighted, and was again, to be fighting 'colds' off by myself.

Then a friend rang. He reminded me that I've been doing

---

[29] There were very few lady doctors then

exercises every day over the past three-four weeks. This was, as he pointed out, unprecedented for me and my body was probably in shock.

OK, OK. I'D OVERDONE IT. AND I'D BEEN FIGHTING OFF AN INFECTION. AND EXERCISING LIKE NEVER BEFORE. OKAY.

But why did I feel like I was going to die? And why was I walking (huh, call that walking?) like a deranged hunchback?

Evening came. I was still in bed. My daughter came home from play rehearsal and our son was still yelling, "I'll do it when I'm ready".[30]

Bladder call again. I waited until it shouted so loud my left arm and shoulder hurt,[31] and then I went.

HURRAH! BINGO, THE ANSWER. MY PERIOD HAD STARTED. WHOOPEE!

Not that I thought I could be pregnant, I didn't. But finally I had my answer to why I felt so shitty. I had suddenly noticed since I stopped working that the first day of my period was hard – a bit painful, tiring and heavy – more heavy than ever before. And the run-up to it, the day before, was tiring as well.

Why, I ask myself, did my period make such a difference? Surely with overdoing it, fighting off a cold, and doing exercise, I had enough reasons? So why did this additional one make such a definite difference?

For me, the difference was all about seeing an end to feeling as I was. I knew my period would only last a couple of days. There was an end to this, not far away. I guess this is what people mean by hope – not just being positive, but really believing that relief is in sight.

Yes, I could try not to overdo it, but where do you stop and draw the line? The problem, as I've said before, is that you have to learn by mistakes – you don't know you've overdone it until you have done it!

Yes, I could fight off infection. But what infection? And how long would it take? Would it go away?

---

[30] It = his homework, of course.
[31] Isn't that weird? It's as though my brain can't cope with more than one message at a time? If I get two, it can't deal sensibly with either.

Yes, I could stop doing exercise. But after three years of physiotherapy I've finally been motivated enough to do it properly and hey presto, it makes a positive difference. It's just knackering that's all.

So, finding a short-term, understandable, reason was brilliant. Just what I needed.

Falling

I do a lot of this. I've been told that I do it because my balance is so bad.

To begin with, I used to fall when something tripped me up – normally an uneven pavement or wayward shoe. I often stumbled because my left foot would not lift up to get over the obstacle. Usually I was moving forwards and that's the way I fell. Gradually my arms' reactions slowed down so they didn't have time to come forward and cushion my fall. I once landed flat on my face and my nose gushed blood. As I told the 'casualty' doctor – about enough blood to fill a small McDonald's coke cup.

After this episode, I learned to slow the rest of me down – so I now walk at a snail's pace. As my balance became more of a problem, I tended to fall over at least once a day. Because I had slowed down my movements generally, I tended to fall quite slowly and always forwards. Tom watched me fall once and said it was like watching slow motion. However, although I tended to have small bumps and bruises all over, none of my falls were really bad since it seemed I had time to avoid hitting most hazards, or at least avoid hitting them with the more vulnerable parts of me.

However, recently, the nature of my falling seems to have changed. I seem to fall less often, maybe once a week, but I fall backwards not forwards. This means that I can't see the hazards around me and my arms can't therefore cushion me from them or direct my fall away from them.

Strangely, I think I fall now even when I'm standing still. I don't know what's going on, all that I know is that I'm hitting my head and my neck more than I used to, plus anything I hit hurts more than it used to.

The other evening I fell upstairs, in the bathroom and, while there were other people in the house, they had music, etc. on too loud to hear me banging on the floor for help. Once I'd calmed down and stopped wailing, I wondered what I would do if I had really hurt myself and couldn't move.

Eventually I got hold of Tom and Alice who were very concerned. I asked them if they could think of a way I could get their attention in such circumstances. Tom thought I should get a rape alarm. Not a bad idea I guess, although I imagine it would deafen me. But, hey, if I needed it, that wouldn't bother me.

I told a friend about this incident and he suggested that I carry my mobile phone with me everywhere I go. So if I had had my mobile with me when I fell in the bathroom, I could have phoned downstairs for help! I guess it's also a good idea because if I'm on my own in the house[32] at least I can phone for outside help. I'll have to make sure that I've got a pocket for the phone in anything I'm wearing or, failing that, wear a cavernous bra that I can stuff it in.

More recently, I came across a leaflet in the doctor's surgery, which was all about an alarm button that you wear like a pendant round your neck. Then I noticed it was from Age Concern and, not being fifty yet (honest), I thought it wasn't for me! So I put the leaflet back. I sat waiting for a bit longer and then, overcoming my pride and prejudice, I picked the leaflet up again. To cut a long story short, I got in touch with Age Concern and I now have a call button pendant and a 'gismo' box, which receives any call signal and phones out for help for you. I feel much better for having it, and my family appears relieved too.

Crutches

Crutches, like the Age Concern call button, were not, in my head, for me. But as it has turned out, my crutches have been a 'life saver'.

A good friend bought me a pair of crutches and suggested I try them. It was very kind of him but I wasn't keen. I associated crutches with broken legs, very often acquired when skiing or doing something else vaguely dangerous, any of which was odious to me. Hence the only way I could imagine using them was to lean on both crutches and swing my legs through them. Far too energetic and hazardous for me. The crutches were also far bigger and more cumbersome than my walking stick – much harder to prop up inconspicuously beside you once you were seated. And anyway, they weren't purple. So they didn't match my wheelchair.

So these were the stupid thought processes that I went through which stopped me using my crutches.

A couple of weeks later I went to Birmingham to take another course of Conductive Education (more about this later in the book). When I met

---

[32] Maggie, the Alsatian, would be here and she'd try to help but having your face licked can only help so much.

one of the 'conductors' I already knew, trusted and believed in, she took one look at me trying to walk with the aid of my (purple) walking stick and said, "You need crutches."

Well, that was it. They got me a set of crutches from their storeroom and showed me how to use them. It was not how I had imagined. I put the right one forward when stepping forward with my left leg, and the left one for my right leg. Just like using two walking sticks. Except I felt much safer because of the arm holds on the crutches.

And I haven't looked back since. I don't care about them being bulky or that they are not purple. They make me feel safe and I can get around by myself. The trouble had been that my walking had got so bad, even with the walking stick, that I needed someone's help to move around at all. Not funny when you suddenly get an urgent need to go to the loo. So, the freedom and independence that the crutches have given me is brilliant.

Is this ME for the REST of my life?

When you've got good health you take it for granted. My Dad used to say, "Look after your health – it's the most important thing you've got." Ironic really, that both his daughters had MS, although he never knew about me. Maybe he does now? Maybe he looks on from above, from another dimension? Who knows?

But it's hard to believe, even when you're not well, that you might never get back to normal again.

People talk about miracle cures – I'm sure I'm not worthy of a miracle, but you never know...

Or maybe it's just my stubbornness or my desire to control things that makes it so difficult for me to accept that I might never get better again. When I speak to someone I haven't seen for a while, I sometimes talk about feeling as though I'm getting better. It's not always a lie; I do occasionally dare to think that I'm feeling a bit more with it, a bit more on top of things. It's a real effort to sustain that though...

Over the page is a painting my good friend did of me. She based it on several photographs. It slightly haunts me actually, but I think it captures the emotional pain, fear and gross uncertainty that MS can promote in me.

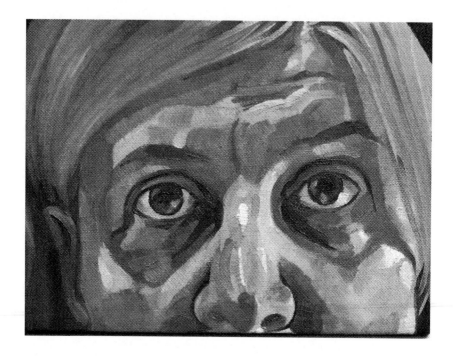

Nearly five years after I gave up work (so now we're at the end of 2003) I came across Dr Hal Huggins' Protocol for Dental Revision. Apparently, he'd taken out the amalgam fillings (metals, particularly mercury), treated the root canals and cleaned out cavities in the gums of over 1,000 MS patients. Many recovered. I had to look into this…

Part 3

Some hope is better than none. Help in foreign parts

These are not my foreign parts; these are more geographical, in the normal sense of the word.

People seem to warn against false hope and I can appreciate some of their meaning. But it seems impossible to me to tell what hope is false until you try it. After all, I assume people aren't lying if they say some people with MS have gained significant benefits from a particular treatment. We're all different, but it might be worth a try. For me, the outlook is seriously black if there is **no** hope.

I've always been open to trying new and different things (hence the "Alternative Therapies" section) and I'm not expecting any one thing to "cure" me. A combination, maybe.

No, seriously, it occurs to me that MS is a very complex condition – each victim is different, new versions of it have been "found" in the last 20 years alone, nobody can predict how it will progress and nobody knows what causes it. I spoke to a University Professor of Neurology about it once, and he said that there was a theory now that a virus causes MS. I also know that I gave my blood to a research programme, being conducted in conjunction with Cambridge University, which is researching whether or not MS is genetic.

The complexity of MS suggests that there will not be one single cause or one single treatment for it. Nor will the causes / treatments be the same for everyone who has MS.

My belief is that a series of factors probably led to my illness – a genetic weakness (because my sister also had MS), environmental elements and stress. My hope is that some combination of treatments will help me. I've done some searching and trying and I know I'll continue until either I don't need help any more, or I run out of options to try.

DENTAL REVISION

Removing Amalgams and More

Out of the blue it came. Our daughter Alice, then 13, was confirmed. I didn't understand this but she did. She said we'd made a promise to God when she was baptised and that her confirmation was the realisation of this promise.

It was a beautiful ceremony with nibbles and a glass of wine afterwards. I met a guy who was feeling very down on his luck and, having conversed for a while, he said he felt much better. And I felt very good about that.

However, the true revelation (gosh, I'm getting biblical) came from my husband, who had been talking to an acquaintance (now a friend!) who is a dentist in Weymouth Street, London. (Round the corner from Harley Street.) This man, David, told Alan about the work of his friend whom he had qualified with and had known for 25-30 years. This friend was Dr. Hal Huggins, which is where I left off at the end of the last section.

Alan called up Huggins' web site (www.hugnet.com) and got a chapter by chapter summary of his book, "Solving the MS Mystery". I read it and ordered the book.

A couple of days later it arrived. I started it straight away, and read it within a couple of weeks. That's good for me (it normally takes months!). I was riveted – it made so much sense. It recognised the urgency of weeing and many other symptoms although I didn't agree that MS people don't sweat – some mornings I wake up saturated! (Later I came across the idea that my body was trying to get rid of the mercury through the skin!) Also, the treatment, which is much more than the dentistry, is designed on an individual basis, so that your diet after Revision works with **your** body chemistry.

Once I finished the book, I was convinced that I should go and have the Dental Revision done – so I phoned up the office and found out the dates that Dr. Huggins was around. Unfortunately, "around" meant when he was at various locations in America and Canada. He doesn't practise in the UK.

I set a provisional date and then started the process of sending the appropriate "bits" of me across the pond to be analysed in advance of the treatment. I got a panoramic X-ray taken of my mouth. (That's great fun, really!) Then I filled out a questionnaire and sent that to Montreal. I got a blood sample taken, centrifuged and frozen and sent it by courier to Colorado Springs. Finally, I got our cleaner to cut off five samples of my hair from the back of my neck and sent that to Chicago.

So, having sorted out all the preliminaries, I'm due to meet Dr. Huggins and colleagues in Montreal. And as I write this, I'm off in five days. Everyone that I've mentioned my trip to has been incredibly supportive, especially my husband and kids.

One of the important things that I have to do is prepare myself mentally. I have to be absolutely clear with myself that there are no positives to my having MS. It sounds weird doesn't it? What could they be? Am I enjoying watching other people working around the house, because I can't? No, don't think so. Do I enjoy not being able to go to work every day? No, I miss the company and the positive "strokes" from clients and colleagues. Although there is some delight (I admit it!) in watching my husband set off to drive up to Leeds (or anywhere else), work for 4 hours and then drive home again late at night as I used to do.

Do I enjoy doing nothing? While there's no pressure from work, I do miss thinking and creating and improving things. I think (see, I do) that's why I did the counselling course and why I'm trying to write this book. It's also why I used to paint – I must get back to that.

Anyway running a house, two teenagers and a husband – you can't call that "doing nothing."

Overall then, I decided that I wanted to give myself permission to get better. There's no overall positive benefit from having MS. Although there are a few positive sides to it – I try and see the positives to keep me sane and try and deal with it – overall, I enjoyed life more before I had the wretched thing. So, I give myself permission to get rid of it.

However, the biggest problem was resolving the, "Don't expect anything so you won't be disappointed", line that Dad was so prone to saying, vs. a quiet confidence that "it was undoubtedly going to work." I wanted to believe that I would, in a short period of time, if not pretty much immediately, see some improvements.

The decision to have my amalgam fillings out (8), my root canal teeth out (6) and my cavitations (3) cleaned out, was easy. It made sense.

- There was a lot of mercury in my amalgam fillings. Authorities in USA declared mercury extremely toxic and regulated it in lakes, rivers, foods (most places, but not your mouth).

- Root canal teeth were shown to be the source of bacteria, many of which were harmful to humans.

- Similarly cavitations, which are air spaces in your gums/bones where extracted teeth used to be, are further sites for toxic materials to grow and/or accumulate.

Where to go to have this done was easy – the protocol I had come to believe in could only be done in North America and from the options, Montreal was the nearest. It also happened to be near Toronto, where I wanted to go to see a friend's dad who was ill.

When to go was easy. The author of the book was only due in Montreal for two weeks in October, or else it was New Year.

Guess what? I kept a diary!

Friday

We flew out in the late afternoon, so there were no nasty get up early times.

Silly things always seem to happen to me – after we checked in, the kids came with me to the loo. It was a disabled one, with basin and loo in one room, with various poles and handles to aid you. I was in my wheelchair (walking for miles in airports does me in – I expect I'm not alone in that!) and I didn't want to put my handbag on the floor because I'd only have to reach down and pick it up later. So, "ah" I thought, thinking myself to be very clever, "I'll put it in the basin." So I did. And I went to the loo. And then got back into my wheelchair and went to wash my hands and rescue my bag. I was mildly amused to see the tap in the washbasin was already in full flow, but less amused when I realised it was flowing straight into the main section of my handbag! I yanked it out and turned it upside-down. Water streamed out, and so did the contents of my handbag.

Once I stopped feeling daft, silly, wet and stupid, I decided to examine the tap more carefully. It had an infrared sensor on the front so it obviously thought my handbag was an unsanitary hand that needed dousing with lots of water. Then, fortunately, I saw the funny side and left the loo in search of family and friends to tell them all about it. I also told the lady at the check-in desk, because she had been very friendly and she thought it was a hoot.

Eventually it was time to get on board and having kissed and waved husband and kids goodbye, off we went. The flight out was good – we left pretty much on time, it took 7 hours, which included watching two films, talking to the steward, who had a brother with MS, and nattering amongst ourselves.

The hotel was fine. I had to fast from 10 p.m. local time because of my blood test the next morning, so we ate quickly and then fell asleep.

Saturday

We went to induction day – we took a cab to the dentist's surgery. Got there at 7.30 am (was OK – it was 12.30 lunchtime to me).

Had 2 test tubes of blood taken. Phew, could eat now – pass me that banana we took from the breakfast room at the hotel.

Then saw lady dentist called Mamon – she looked at my teeth and declared "ugh," they were mucky and needed cleaning, then she took casts and electrical readings from my amalgams. "You've got a battery in your mouth," she said. Then Dr Benoit joined us. Very soon after that I saw someone was behind him – and then I saw Huggins grinning over his shoulder – it was hard to talk while sitting in the dentist's chair with various obstacles in my mouth!

Then consulted with Huggins, who it was great to meet after reading his book, talking on the phone and hearing the dentist dad talk about him. He started off by saying he "selfishly" wanted my root canal teeth! This was because he was hoping to conduct some more research on samples of ground down root canal teeth. Unfortunately, the samples that he did have were thrown away by a hotel maid. I said he was welcome to them since it didn't bother me what happened to them once they had left my mouth.

He also decided that I must be strong, otherwise I'd be laid out by all the stuff in my mouth. Finally, I thought, someone who understands.

He asked me what my 3 wishes were – I said to walk properly (no stick, let alone a wheelchair), to chase my son round the garden (I'm not sure I could have done this without MS) and catch him (some hope, he's 16!)

Also to get my right hand back so I can type better, write and, importantly, paint again.

Not having a constant battle to get a comfortable temperature would also be good. I've pretty much learnt how to deal with hot/cold during the day, but at night time it's more of a problem. There I am, lying there in the middle of the night, trying to keep my right hand, arm and shoulder warm, and my left leg warm (especially the knee which is freezing) while at the same time, making sure my left arm and right leg are not too hot. Think that "Twister" can be difficult? Try organising all your limbs as above! At least it's only me playing. Although I wonder sometimes...

Maybe my neurological consultant in London would be interested if I had a MRI scan after treatment to see if there are any noticeable changes? However, MRI scans are not cheap, and who knows if this treatment reduces the plaques (the debris) anyway? Maybe other people have tried to find evidence of change? I think there is some, but not from a MRI scan. Regardless, HH thinks plaques are an artefact. Maybe that's convenient? Despite all this, I found I liked HH more than I thought I would.

Sunday
Had Swedish massage – lovely.

Going into the dentists again – to get my teeth cleaned. They had a tube that squirted lots of water into your mouth and then another tube to suck it all out again. During all the pressure hosing there was also sandblasting using baking soda. It took a long time – because my teeth were very stained (they'd not been cleaned for three years). Glad when it stopped. Noticed no "rinse and spit" apparatus next to the dentist's chair, they used all the suction. So, as my husband observed, it seems that the Brits spit while the Canadians hoover.

Monday
Had ECG this morning – very quick. Medical centre – like a tall shopping centre, but all medical – conventional and alternative. Then we went onto the roof of the hotel where there were great views since we were on the 21st floor. And then we went to visit the Cranial Osteopath. Found him through Gez. The guy, called Alain, was very interested

in meeting one of Gez's patients and in HH's work. He spent time balancing out the back of my head (like wood he said, I've heard that before) and the front forehead (like wet clay he said – that's a new one). I would guess that that was about my gut (primitive brain) reaction to tomorrow's dentistry being quite scared, while consciously my thinking brain is quite rational and relaxed about it – I'm sort of looking forward to it – especially the benefits I expect from it.

He also balanced out my jaw – where it articulates with the bone at its top (the skull bit). As I'll have my mouth open for up to 8 hours[1] tomorrow, I wanted to start with my jaw as well aligned as I could!

He and I are looking forward to how I am next week when I go to see him again.

Tuesday

The long awaited surgery day. I woke up in a bit of a tearful tizz. What if it didn't work? What if it hurt? A lot? All the elements of the, "Don't expect too much (anything?)" vs. "You've got to believe for it to work," debate reared their ugly heads. Still, we had to get there so early (7.15 am – don't these Canadians ever sleep?) I didn't really have time to dwell on it. Everybody was there – raring to go. By then I was quite happy – after all, this is what I came for.

I started with the anaesthetist, a super guy – I never caught his name – it was very French – I couldn't say it, let alone remember it. He had read my form, knew about the Amantadine and Beta Interferon and that I said I would give up smoking at the end of September. I confessed that I'd had a couple the day before (oh, that's what she was doing on the roof) and just a few before that. Much to my delight he didn't have a go at me – it was more like he understood that a girl's got to have a fag now and then.

Anyway, once the needle was in my arm, I was quickly off. What do they put in those things? And why do you have to be ill before you get some? It was conscious sedation (a form of valium I think) and it was fabulous. I was drifting about, very pleasurably, most of the time.

I went to the loo twice during my 8-hour stint in the chair – I remember walking there and performing quite clearly. I also have some memory of someone grabbing a tooth and pulling and twisting it. This didn't last long, I closed down before I saw or knew anything else. It

[1] "What's new?" I heard someone say!

was almost as though I didn't want to spy on whoever was doing the "business."

And so the day whizzed by.

Wednesday

Guess what? I could rest today. So I did. I stayed in bed. There were highlights to the day though:

- In the morning, I could take my partial dentures out, and swill with warm salt water around my mouth – well, I had to take the water into my mouth, and then turn my head from side to side, like one of those manic looking dogs you see on the back shelf of cars. And no spitting. That would dislodge the blood clots that were forming where the root canal teeth (6, remember) had been.
- In the afternoon, the small magnet I had on each cheek came off. This meant my carer could no longer threaten to leave me attached by the magnets to the fridge door.
- Just to punctuate the day and keep my carer on his toes, I took painkillers, homeopathic and conventional, whenever I could.
- And, if all that wasn't riveting enough, the real highlight was tea. This was blended roast beef and baked potato. Ever tried to drink a savoury milk shake?

Thursday

I was quite getting into this blended food now. Porridge was good, scrambled egg too.

This was my first class day – we had to go to a hotel room and watch an hour or so of video before lunch (sorry about the noise of the blender) and then have a seminar with Dr. Huggins in the afternoon.

Today's topic was "miscellaneous". It was a bit puzzling, since it picked up many subjects that had been covered in previous days. (He runs a four-day topic course, which I was told you could join on any day – trust me to start at the end!) But I was OK.

Friday

Was wiped out from yesterday, so the nurse came up to my room to take my blood sample. Also watched the requisite tape from my bed, and then lunch (it's amazing what will pass as lunch…)

Went down to the conference room after slurping. Today's topic was Carbohydrate Metabolism.

We met some people from the Huggins team on the way to the conference room; they both said how good I looked. When we got into the lift alone, I looked at the mirrored wall and both Nino and I said together, "God, you/I must have looked shit!"

Saturday

Another early get up – we had to be at the dentist's by 9.00. We almost were, and I saw Dr. Huggins, who had the results of yesterday's blood sample. He was very pleased. He thinks it will take a while for me to get better, though. I think this is because my BUN, albumin and total protein are low. These all went down after the dental revision – I'm not sure why. Need more protein?

I've noticed that I move a little more freely now, with more confidence perhaps. Hooray! I also don't seem to have to go to the loo as often, although it's still pretty urgent when I feel the need. It's hard to believe I spent most of my pre-MS life being like a camel.

Sunday

Today was the first total rest day we've had. I've been looking forward to today since we got here. I've certainly done more here than I would have done at home. To be blunt, I'm knackered. Slept quite a bit in the morning then got very introspective and emotional from about lunchtime onwards. This wasn't good, especially since it was my carer's birthday. And I forgot. Oops.

Finally, that evening, life got better and we had a take-away Chinese, carefully chosen, I thought, to avoid the things I'm not allowed. Anyway, we didn't eat much. Which was just as well, as my stomach started to hurt when I was in bed. I still slept though and nothing else happened. We threw the rest of the food away. We watched Double Jeopardy on VCR.

Monday

This is my last day of classes and although I enjoy them, I'm glad to have completed another part of the process. We said goodbye to Robbie and Dwayne (paediatrician) who had their two kids (2 and 8) plus nanny, with them. I tried to work out what I would have done if I'd come here when the kids were younger – I don't know.

Said goodbye to a few others who were in this "class", and picked up a list of everyone's contact details. Everyone seemed much more open, fun and approachable than before – maybe illness turns you inward.

I felt a bit better again today. Improvements seem to be very subtle. A tiny bit better writing and slightly more confidence standing and walking. I also seem to be going to the loo less often, although with a similar sense of urgency. Maybe I'm even sleeping a bit better.

Tuesday

Went back to see the cranial osteopath, Alain, today. It was fun. I think he genuinely felt I had changed – I asked him what my head felt like now – it had been wood and clay. He said it felt softer now, like Jell-O! He also talked about my jaw being wonky and tried to straighten it out, a bit at least. He gave me a card with the areas for the cranial lady to work on when I get back and it was a very warm-hearted, almost sad, goodbye. Overall though, I was very happy. We had ventured out without a wheelchair – it felt like progress.

Driving back to the hotel in the cab, it was beautiful weather – crisp, bright, sunny and very welcoming. We decided we'd go visit old Montreal this afternoon, so we did. The wheelchair came with us, since we wanted to be able to cover some ground since the stories we were told made me think it was going to be like Covent Garden at home. We started at their Notre Dame, an RC Cathedral. Nino pushed me around, once I'd got up the ramp. It was very fresh and clean looking (typical of Montreal) with many candles and figures on the walls. We lit one for Nino's Dad. I thought about lighting one for Mum, Dad and Judy, but they've gone. It seemed right to light one for someone who was still with us but needs help and support to make the most of his time left (apparently 18 months to 2 years). Gosh, this Dental Revision is very sobering.

Being sober is something I'll have to get used to. Not allowed alcohol you see, a bit of red wine maybe, but not a lot. In fact white wine is better apparently.

Nino pushed me round some streets of old Montreal and we passed many wine bars, coffee places and pubs. I couldn't go in any of them (not allowed caffeine either) and it made me realise the kind of places where I normally spent my life. So Nino kept pushing, making me do the occasional wheelie, and as it got dark we decided to go "home" as it was getting fairly cold! So we found a cab, which was an estate car and so big enough to take our chariot, and went back.

Looking back on it now, I think if I went back I would stop and get a de-caffeinated coffee and a glass of wine at one, or maybe two, of the places we passed. But it was all so new to me, and Nino was driving so fast (bless) that we were confined to peering in the windows of various art galleries, picking out the pictures we'd like.

Wednesday

We went back to the dental surgery to square up my bill. We are flying back home to Heathrow tomorrow evening, so today is definitely goodbye to all the friends we made at Dr. Benoir's. (I never thought I'd say that about a Dentist's Surgery!) It was quite sad and we spent hours there just hanging about! I settled up, tested the pH of my urine, bought some Huggins books and just sat at Anna's desk, causing trouble. I had forgotten what a double act Nino and I could be but during this trip we were reborn! So I don't forget (how could I?):

Anna – nominally the receptionist, but really she ran the place. She and Nino had great fun as she was of Italian heritage too. Her husband is a chef, and I invited them to stay with us in London if…

Mamon – she did a lot of my dental work. She cleaned me up to start with and changed my amalgam fillings. I was very comfortable with her, and felt safe.

Carl Benoir – the main man. According to Nino, Carl did the 6 extractions, although he couldn't bear to look. Nino, that is.

Caroline – I had spoken to her on the phone before arriving when she had sorted out the finances. She did a bit of the dental work for me – mainly sanding off a sharp bit of my bottom denture. She was really sweet and giggled a lot.

Stephanie – had only been working at the practice for one week. She was very tall and slim, and she told Nino that she had a degree in Media Studies. There a bond was made! E-mails are flowing now!

Then there was the nurse, and the ladies that did the massage. Plus, not forgetting the hotel staff, who let us change rooms after the first night and let us use a small table from the roof as a shower seat!

All in all, it worked pretty well. It was a very enjoyable adventure!

Thursday

Our very last day – pack up time. Nino packed me up, and all his books! We got an extension at the hotel – paid for another night because it just wasn't worth the hassle of sitting around for 3-4 hours before a long haul flight. The trip home was uneventful, but good. We had the wind behind us, so although we left late, we landed slightly early.

Friday

And there they were – Alan and Alice – the latter was very sleepy (it was 7.30 a.m.!) Tom was so sleepy; he never made it out of the car!

We had McDonald's on the way home and then started the real-life saga of what I could eat and, a longer list, what I couldn't. I had an egg McMuffin – but I could only eat the egg! Still, never mind – it feels like it's already worth it!

When I had time to think about it, I certainly felt better than before I went to Montreal. Before my adventure, my walking, balance, urgency of urinating, the sensations in my right hand and my energy levels were all much worse. I remember feeling like I was sliding into a large black pit. It was funnel shaped – steep sloping sides leading to an inescapable vertical tube, that you couldn't see inside of.

After Montreal I felt that the funnel was still there but that someone had placed friendly ladders all around the inside of it. At least now I had a chance of climbing out. However slowly.

The first thing to do was to consolidate my diet, both in my head and with my family.

My diet, which was permanent:
• nothing out of the sea (i.e. fish, shellfish, salt).
• no bread (allergy to gluten already established via blood test).

- limited intake of heavy carbohydrates (wheat, potato, rice and corn).
- no pork (I miss bacon!)
- no caffeine (tea as well as coffee).
- very limited alcohol – only a small glass of wine, at most. White is better than red, although I prefer red. Of course!

My conclusion about the Dental Revision was positive when I first got home. I had begun to feel better about a week after the dental surgery. I certainly became more confident and walked without a wheelchair and, sometimes, without a stick.

Two and a Half Months Later

I have not written for this time because I concentrated on typing up the notes from HH's talks. Actually the real truth is that there weren't that many notes and that Christmas, lethargy and a broken Internet connection, all distracted me.

My husband Alan commented very soon after I got home that I seemed to have more energy than before I went to Canada. And that has stayed with me – it's still not as easy to do stuff as it was before MS but I can keep awake and with it for longer than before I went. (I need shorthand for "before I went"– think it'll be BDR – Before Dental Revision). Some days my balance is better and so is my walking but I still need a stick. In fact, I've progressed to having a "downstairs" stick and an "upstairs" one as well – because a stick doesn't help with the stairs – it just stops me grabbing on to the banister and walls as I go up, or down.

Having said that, there has been a few days – most recently – when I've raced up the stairs. Well, I say raced, I mean quick for me!

Going to the loo less often has stayed with me. In fact, I think I was getting back to "normal" in this regard, with night time forays down to once, at most twice, and even sometimes I slept straight through – 8 or 9 hours worth – now there's bladder control!

Then I did one of the detox things – had a "cocoon"[2] bath and after that I started going to the loo more often again. Need to do another? Don't think so, because it was so frightening to find that my legs would not move when I stayed in the bath just for two minutes beyond the 20 minute maximum that HH had recommended. Besides that, sweating, which the cocoon bath encourages, has never been difficult for me! Most nights I have

---

[2] This is lying in a bath, at body temperature, with a large towel, also dunked in the bath water, covering you from head to toe. So you are surrounded by heat.

to turn my saturated pillow over at least once after I've got out of bed and gone to the loo because the wet/damp has got too cold in my absence. What a faff, as my mum would say!

But I did do the C flush that HH recommended. Apart from the gory detail (which I will try to keep down to a bare minimum) this is worth telling because it's so odd! Firstly, you need some Vitamin C in the form of sodium ascorbate. I found this difficult in the UK (and had it sent from Colorado) because all I could find was Vitamin C in the form of ascorbic acid – not to be used according to HH. And in view of where it was going, I wasn't going to risk it! Anyway, then you put a teaspoon in 4oz water and drink it down in one go. Twenty minutes later, use a kitchen timer that rings when your time is up (should have done that for the cocoon bath!) do the same thing again. Keep going until diarrhoea sets in. Very attractive. Keep near a loo. Preferably your own.

It took about 6 goes to achieve "lift off" for me – so about 1 hour 40 minutes! Unlike normal diarrhoea, it stopped quite quickly and didn't involve any stomach ache or after effects. According to HH you're supposed to do this once a week for 3 weeks, stop for a week, then another 3-week stint. Every time you do it you're supposed to drink 'friendly bacteria' afterwards – you know the type, they're advertised on the telly. The C flush is supposed to get rid of unfriendly bacteria and parasites and help you to digest your food better. I'm not sure how often you are supposed to do this – it can't be that often, otherwise you'd flush yourself down the loo! I must find out.

Overall, I think that while I did feel better when I first got home, I then fairly steadily slid back again, although I still feel better than I did before the dental surgery.

Another Two and a Half Months Later

I must send a blood test through to Colorado for an up-date. Nothing else has really changed – I still feel better than before I left for Montreal last September, but I still need my stick and I haven't even been in the garden at all, never mind chased Tom around it!

Blood Test Up-date

This time instead of sending the blood to Colorado, I had the test done here, under Hugginite instructions, and sent the results to the States. Then

I spoke to Elisa on the phone. She gave me some pointers and wants me to do another blood test and hair analysis in a couple of months time. In the meantime, the pointers were:

- Calcium is still a problem for me and I wonder where on earth it all comes from. I mean, I really don't stuff my face with cheese and milk! I'm reminded of the distinction between calcium in the blood and calcium in the bones. Anyway cheese now has to be an infrequent treat for me, at most.
- I also have to reduce my grain intake. I've avoided wheat for several years because of the gluten, but now I'm looking at no grains at all. I need to find out the definition of grain[3]. Think it means no porridge in the mornings. Well, not every morning, like I do now!
- More protein is required. So, more eggs and meat – beef, lamb, chicken and turkey – well chewed. Elisa said to eat protein twice a day, at least 3/4 times a week.
- I need to eat more salt too.
- I have to return to taking my vitamin A drops. I stopped because they were a 'faff' and tasted disgusting; but, in for a penny...
- I have to try and do the detox bath – the cocoon that I had trouble with before. Apparently starting with a couple of minutes in the cocoon is better (rather than the 22 minutes that ended up with my legs simply not working). I need to do this 2/3 times a week and shower immediately afterwards in order to wash the toxins that I've sweated out of my system away.
- Elisa also said that intravenous vitamin C would help. There has to be nothing else in solution with it and it has to take three and a half – four hours to drip through. Ideally this should be done once a month. I need to phone my GP and get a protocol/prescription from the States. In the meantime, I could possibly take more vitamin C tablets?

It interests me how my attitude to all these instructions has changed since I had the Dental Revision work done over nine months ago. Having committed to it then, it seems stupid not to continue with it in good faith now. I believed in it then, I need to believe in it again. OK, the effect wore off as soon as I got home – but the effect was there. Just like my walking was better after I'd been to Birmingham (to be conductively educated) but

---

[3] I've decided not to worry about grain – I can't find a consistent definition. And anyway, I'll be living off fresh air if I exclude any more!

soon declined once I was home. And the same happened when I returned from Holland (to have my free radicals magnetised away).

What is going on? It can't be the house or the animals in it because I didn't improve when we stayed for a few days at a hotel across New Year. Maybe a few days isn't long enough?

Much later

I wish I'd never had the cocoon bath – I was relying on Alan to time 20 minutes, but he didn't believe how key 20 (NOT 22) was,[4] and ended up hauling me out of the bath. He complained his back hurt while I crumpled onto the floor since my legs did not work at all.

Anyway, forget the stick, now I need crutches and I'm feeling very angry and pissed off. Best shut up for a while.

[4] Got distracted by something on the TV – golf probably.

ELIMINATING FREE RADICALS

The Essaïdi Aqua Tilis Therapy

Believe it or not, my oldest friend (I don't mean she's ancient, I mean we've known each other since we were six) called and suggested I try this treatment NOW.

Although I had gone through the Dental Revision six months ago, I felt that maybe that was only part of the answer, so I was ready to try the treatment in Holland.

So at the end of March off I went. Another adventure!

I knew the treatment had something to do with water. I imagined, because I had nothing else to base my thoughts on, that it involved me floating in a tank! Anyway, I didn't mind, since I was going to spend a week with my old mate!

The first thing was to get to her. This involved going to Stanstead airport and getting a short flight across to Eindhoven. Sounds easy, doesn't it?

We got to the airport just as check-in was about to close. Our delay was due to an accident on the motorway. Never mind, the staff decided to let me onto the plane. So, I checked in and kissed goodbye to husband, son and daughter, then a staff lady wheeled me off.

My temporary carer was, like me, called Sue. And another coincidence, her family came from, and still lived in, a part of Yorkshire that was the same as my mum originated from. I found all this out because we spent quite a bit of time together nattering – the flight was delayed!

As it turned out, the flight was delayed by three hours in the end. However, I think that some of this time was due to me. Being in a wheelchair, I had to wait for "assistance" to board the plane. The flight was called, the other passengers filed on and I was left sitting at the gate waiting. Eventually the assistance arrived, comprising one man and one woman. They seemed to be having a great natter and insisted on taking me back to the main terminal on the monorail, so we could get the right monorail out to the right aircraft. It was true that our aircraft had changed due to a cracked windscreen and anyway, what could I do?

I finally got wheeled out to the correct aircraft and had to climb (very slowly) the stairs (a shame that, I was promised a hoist up!). I felt bad when

I got inside – the whole plane was seated, ready and staring daggers in my direction. Fortunately, I got help into my seat at the front from the hostess. She told me not to worry – it wasn't my fault. However, I felt eyes searing into the back of my head for a while.

During the short flight, another little detail conspired against us. Our destination, Eindhoven airport, was closed because we left so late, so we were going to land in Dusseldorf! Not just wrong city, but wrong country! However, even I'm enough of a European to know that Holland and Germany are next to each other!

Well, what a commotion that all caused. Whoever said the English don't complain? They did.

Nonetheless we landed in Dusseldorf and went through German customs with our bags. They were going to get us to Eindhoven by coach. Sitting outside Dusseldorf airport I got talking to a guy who worked there and had been responsible for ordering the coaches that would take us to Eindhoven. His English was very good, and we passed the time quite congenially – me in my wheelchair, and him crouched down beside it. Eventually the coaches appeared, but I couldn't step up into even the smallest – a big minibus. So, he carried me up. At the same time he told two other guys who were travelling with us to look after my case and wheelchair, which had to go into another coach.

Anyway, two hours later we pulled up in Eindhoven airport. Only one o'clock in the morning!

The two guys unloaded my case and 'chair and waited with me until my (oldest) friend arrived. I noticed that both the guys were wearing 'Aston Martin' jackets. It turned out that they only worked for and demonstrated my most favourite car ever! They were really impressed that I knew what the marque was.

Anyway, then my friend arrived at about one thirty in the morning and the chaps went off on their way. Lizzie and I went to the hotel and I slept like a log. Then came the rude awakening – off to have the first treatment. I know my appointment was 11 that morning, but after the excursions of the night before, I was truly blitzed.

Lizzie drove us to the Essaïdi Centre. It was in the middle of a countrified area and was a very pleasant place to be.

We felt very much at ease there since Lizzie had been there before. We went in to meet Mr. Essaïdi. He spoke seven languages. This did not include English so his daughter, Hannah, translated for us (although Lizzie speaks

Dutch, so some of it was through her). I started by mentioning the Dental Revision I'd been through. Mr. Essaïdi said that I need not have bothered, which put my back up a bit. But I made myself relax and not worry about that. I kept listening and had the treatment explained to me: apparently at great length because I kept asking questions – well, I wanted to know!

I won't relate it all because I'm not sure I can remember it all and anyway, he explains it better! The main theory was that we have free radicals (which are electrically charged neutrons that have escaped from their atoms) in our body and they can cause a lot of damage. He listed a lot of ailments that they cause which ranged from psoriasis to cancer and included MS. The treatment they offered involved removing some (all?) free radicals from the body. They did this by heating you up to make you sweat and bring the particles to the surface of your skin. They then used electro-magnets to draw the free radical particles away from you. This was done inside a pyramid-shaped cabin that had the magnets outside of it.

The cabin was lined with mirrors. Since you go in naked you have to be fairly comfortable with your shape, or very short-sighted! What I found weird was seeing my face turn purple as the treatment progressed. It comprised:

- I got on to a flat plastic-covered bed
- and lay on my back for 5 minutes while the temperature increased quickly to HOT
- then I turned over, for another "hot" five minutes
- then I got scrubbed down, and hosed with warm water. This is the part that Lizzie, having kept cooler by sitting in a bath in the cabin, really enjoyed. "Ooh" she said, "it's just like washing a car". The idea is to get rid of any free radicals still on the skin.
- and then the whole process got repeated.

In total, I got heated up for 20 minutes. They took me up to 55 degrees centigrade. There is an intercom in the cabin, so we stayed "in touch" with the controller all the time. 55 was a bit hot for me, so I was at 53-54 most of the time. But I was pleasantly surprised how enjoyable the whole process was. Especially since I typically find heat uncomfortable (I simply don't work!). However, I think the timing is key. You're heated up for only 20 minutes, and that comprises short bursts of 5 minutes. 20 minutes was the same time period that was recommended by HH (above). Interestingly, HH and Essaïdi's approach had quite a few similarities. I must tell HH the next time I speak to him.

The whole process, including getting undressed, sitting around to cool down after the cabin experience and then getting dressed again took about two hours. This comprised one treatment. Five treatments are recommended for a course of therapy. One treatment a day.

I was over in Eindhoven for a week, so I had 2 days of treatments, the weekend to rest and then the three other treatments. Lizzie and I got into a wonderful routine of going to the Centre at 11 o'clock, getting back to the hotel anywhere between 4 and 6, immediately having a meal,[5] and then crashing back in our room. We'd fall asleep at about 9 or 10. Or midnight, if we were talking, which we did quite a lot!

After the final treatment I underwent a 'sweat test'. They put me into a sunbed, heated me up for about 8 minutes and then collected my sweat in a pipette and sent it off for analysis, which was going to take a fortnight.

I had one final meeting with Essaïdi to review how I was and how all the treatment had gone. It was a very amiable session, especially since he said he thought I wouldn't get any worse. Interestingly, he, like HH, thought unconventionally about the plaques that you typically get with MS. He thought they were accumulations of excess calcium, not the debris left after the immune system had been to war on your nerve cells. I'm sure I'm over simplifying what he said but I know it was different to what I've heard before.

It was a great week – a lot of fun and very restful. The only downside to it was my having to drink 30 ml of "tonic" four times a day. Honestly, it was disgusting. The worst thing I've ever tasted in all my life. I asked Mr Essaïdi what it was. He said it was all herbs, waved a packet of one of them at me and told me it was good for me. To start with I protested; how could something that tasted so awful, be good for me? Surely my body wouldn't let something that was good for us taste so bad? Undeterred, he insisted it would give me more energy and that I should carry on with it. So I did. I even took some home, because I have to admit I did seem to have a bit more energy. I even kept forgetting to take the Amantadine tablets because I didn't experience the energy "lows" that would remind me to take one.

However, at four times a day my supply didn't last long. I'll have to get my head around getting some more. It'll take some organising because

---

[5] Nearly always at the very good restaurant attached to the hotel, served by very charming staff, some of whom were quite hunky! Lizzie called our favourite waiter "cutie pie", and he was a really nice guy (there's a surprise) who was hoping to study psychology.

Essaïdi doesn't ship it, so I'm reliant on my old friend to get it across to me somehow.

So, how did I feel when I got home? I felt quite rested and relaxed, and could walk slightly better. Unfortunately, we had already arranged to have a week on a narrow boat. Alice and Tom had one friend each, so there were six of us. It was a very good week, everyone got on and helped. The reason I say unfortunately was that it was hard to practice walking on the boat – not much room and it was, by definition, narrow! Hence it was too easy to hold on to something rather than just walk free form. However, I was thankful for the walls since we were floating and so I wasn't that stable! I could have walked on shore, I hear you say, but getting off the boat was a bit of a procedure and the towpath wasn't exactly level and easy to practice on.

The week after we returned from the boat I got my sweat analysis results. Lizzie told me a summary: I didn't have cancer[6] or a virus, and I was detoxing some substances in my sweat that don't normally come out until someone has had more than a couple of treatments. Maybe HH had given me a head start? Or, my habitual nocturnal clamminess had?

Lizzie also told me that the analysis showed I had too much calcium[7] in my sweat, and that I needed to take more Magnesium[8] and Vitamin D. The Magnesium had to be Mg++ and taking Calcium++ would also be good. This isn't totally alien to me,[9] but I don't pretend to totally understand it. Anyway, this is something else I need to get my head around.

[6] That was good news for me but it must have brought back memories for Lizzie because she'd gone with her Mum, who had cancer, to Essaïdi a while ago. Unfortunately she had died about a year before my trip.
[7] But the wrong type of Calcium. This is another similarity with HH who also said I had enough calcium in my system to turn to stone: but that it was the wrong type. I needed biological calcium not the inert calcium that I had since my body couldn't use the latter. HH reckoned that one of the best sources of biological calcium was, wait for it, lettuce.
[8] Another similarity. Both Essaïdi and HH believed that there is a strong relationship between calcium and magnesium and that you had to take more of the latter to reduce the former.
[9] Since I did chemistry and biology A level, albeit a long time ago!

CONDUCTIVE EDUCATION

A good friend (in fact, the same one that I mentioned at the beginning of the book) brought me an article that she'd saved from the Guardian. Nicky Broyd, a journalist who had unfortunately been diagnosed with relapsing remitting MS five years previously, wrote it. She had attended a two-week course of 'conductive therapy' at the National Institute of Conductive Education in Birmingham. The descriptions of her experiences, and what she said about the value of the course, sparked off my interest in pursuing NICE therapy.

The article said that the main institute is the Petö in Budapest. This interested me too, since we had had a nanny from Slovenia, who had trained as a physiotherapist there and whose approach to physio was quite different to that which I'd experienced in the UK. She used to help with my left leg and foot – and it really did make them more mobile. Her approach centred on moving my limbs to remind my brain of what certain movements felt like. This feedback route, together with some degree of brain control to make my limbs move, really did help. Unfortunately, this lady left us quite a few years ago.

Thinking about it, I realise that Birmingham isn't exactly foreign parts. However, I remember from research days that whenever we did projects which included going to Birmingham, we always found a slightly different response there. For example, we were doing the original work for the Silentnight beds 'hippo and duck' campaign, and I was talking to a group of women. We had got to beds in general and the group agreed that drawers in a double bed were OK but not necessary for storage or strength. Then, a previously fairly quiet lady said:

"Er, well, yuv obviously never made luv to a prop forward".

The group thought about this! Then another inquisitive lady pondered:

"Yeah, but don't it make yer drawers rattle?"

Well. This just about finished us all off!

Another time we were working for a shoe company and were discussing the merits, or otherwise, of leather shoes. We'd got to the idea that if leather shoes became wet, then your feet tended to get wet too. And then a lady said, rather ponderously,

"Well, it's funny i'nt it, 'cos cows don't leak."

Sorry. Back to NICE. I learnt later that there are degree courses for conductors in the U.K. Apparently Warwick University has one, as does the University of Wolverhampton. Their training covers a whole range of disciplines, including neurology, disability, physiology, psychology, education, teaching, rehabilitation and motor learning.

I also found a definition: "Conductive Education is a form of special education and rehabilitation for children and adults with motor disorders. It is appropriate for conditions where disease or damage to the central nervous system affects a person's ability to control movement. In childhood these conditions include cerebral palsy and dyspraxia, and in adulthood, Parkinson's disease, multiple sclerosis, cerebral palsy and those who have had a stroke or head injury."

I was very interested and so I phoned up, and they sent me some information, plus a questionnaire about me. I filled in all the details of my condition and posted it off pretty quick since I couldn't see the point of delaying.

Shortly afterwards my husband and I went to Birmingham to see the NICE people for an initial consultation. They told me that they couldn't cure me; well, I wasn't expecting them to do that, I was hoping they would help me move around better. They also said that they did not recommend any exercises for after the course. As you can imagine, that was music to my ears! They said quite simply that they thought that for MS if you couldn't do something when you were with them, then you wouldn't be able to do it with exercise later. We'll see, maybe I didn't understand that right?

We were there for an hour during which two conductors put me through my paces (well, sort of). They filmed me moving around. After about half an hour they quickly summarised the workings (or otherwise) of my body.

Of course, I knew some of the details already, but there were some fascinating snippets that were new to me. I knew that my main problems were my left leg and right arm, plus that I was using my right leg to compensate, and that balance was a big problem. However, I didn't realise that my arms worked independently, not as a unit, like they're supposed to. The conductors said they could work on the arms to stop them becoming more of a problem in the future.

They also focussed on the fact that I use my torso, especially my shoulders, to move around, when other parts of me should be doing the work and would be more effective. That is, my legs! And, particularly, my HIPS.

They also said that I seem to be spending a lot of time and energy chasing round my centre of balance, and not quite finding it.

Overall though, they were incredibly positive. They told me my range of movement was good, and most importantly, THEY COULD HELP ME improve it. Plus, they thought that more efficient movement would reduce the fatigue I experience.

It all sounded brilliant. I'd love to be able to walk like a 'normal' person, plus go up stairs without needing a mini-crane to haul my legs up. I would also love to be able to write and type like I used to.

So I booked onto the next available course.

My NICE trip 28.6.04.

Off I went on the start of my two-week (except weekends) course. I had arranged four 'shifts' of helpers – good souls who could give me 3-4 days each.

Suze, a lady who I had worked with for many years, drove me up to Birmingham on Sunday night. She managed to cram my wheelchair into the back of her Audi TT (with the back seats down) and off we went. We checked into the hotel, had a bite to eat from room service and fell asleep.

On Monday, we got to the centre just before ten and discovered that there were four of us in the class and we all had MS. One other lady, Kate, was like me – she could stand upright, and walked with help – while the other two, Jackie and Margaret, were more bound to their wheelchairs. Two 'conductors,' Mel (English) and Aggy (Hungarian), the same two that were at my initial consultation, took the two-hour session on Monday and then again on Tuesday. Thereafter we had a mix of conductors taking each session. Normally Aggy was there plus another conductor. The new conductors were all Hungarian, with amazingly good English, especially considering the specialised area they were dealing with.

All four of us 'participants' were extremely impressed by the knowledge, commitment and approachability of the conductors. They really were more helpful and effective than any other therapist that any of us had met before.

We spent most of the sessions lying down on 'beds'. These were fairly narrow wooden slatted platforms with a thin foam covering. Apparently in Hungary participants lie directly on the slats, which just goes to show how 'soft' we Brits are! It's all designed to provide feedback to the brain and body while you move it around in different positions. This is important since we needed to learn what various sensations meant, because the nerves that we used pre-MS were often not functioning anymore. So the brain had to find new pathways to use.

So, for example, we all began by trying to lie straight. I say 'trying to' because none of us got this right from the outset. This was a fundamental part of learning what different sensations meant – we could lift our heads and look to see where our feet were – but that was only part of the process, and kind of cheating, because the ultimate point was to FEEL it.

We were lying down because it was safer than standing, but we simulated standing – we had to keep our feet flexed up.

Being in wheelchairs, Jackie and Margaret always first had to get themselves 'transferred' from the chairs to the 'beds'. This was very clever and involved a board which, once they were on it, they could slide across to move from one to the other. Across the span of the ten sessions, both of them became very adept at this and many other things.

By the final day, both Jackie and Margaret stood up. People helped them and they had bars they could lean on but they did a fair amount of the work themselves and, importantly, they were standing. The wide-mouthed grins and smiles said it all – they hadn't experienced that view for years.

Kate and I concentrated on walking. In particular, we had to "walk the ladder". This was hard, since with the ladder lying on the floor, we had to lift our legs up to get over each step. It was quite a challenge – in the end, it felt a bit like walking the plank! But we knew it was good for us and the round of applause when we did it was fun.

We practised going upstairs (and coming down again!) which involved using some of the movements we had done when we were lying down.

We were encouraged to do fine movements, including writing, co-ordinating our arms together, breathing, and a lot more.

Throughout the whole course there was an emphasis on repeating actions while concentrating and being very aware of the feedback sensations that the movements resulted in. Hopefully, this process of learning would lead to you moving without thinking so that you could, eventually, move automatically.

Automatic or not, another primary aim was to move more effectively and therefore decrease fatigue.

Active resting[10] was also suggested as a response to feeling tired.

Overall, for me, it was great. I walked and moved more easily, including stepping into the (high) car instead of falling onto the seat bum first and then needing to swing/lift my legs round. Unfortunately, the benefits disappeared after a weekend at home.

Nevertheless, I went back for a one week course in February 2005. The improvement wasn't as noticeable this time, although I was worse to start with by then.

However, I am now willing to exercise at home because I know that there were very tangible benefits from the first course straight away/in a short time. I've got a video from the first session which I'm going to show my carer – she only comes round twice a week, but that'll be a start.

---

[10] That is, lying or sitting down and doing something – reading, for example!

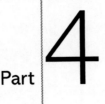

Another year on

DISABLED DRIVING

Fortunately, I didn't get into trouble for not telling the DVLC about the MS earlier.

I assume that since apparently most people with MS aren't aware that they have to inform the DVLC about their condition, then my details will go on record and the Medical Department will investigate my fitness to drive.

I decided to get a professional's opinion of my driving and my car. I wanted to know:

- Will I have to get my Mini adapted for driving?
- If so, will it be something that can be fixed, and then easily taken off again?
- Will I have to get rid of the Mini?[1]

Driving Assessment

This was in Welwyn Garden City (at least I'm getting closer to home!) and Alan, my husband, drove me up there in my beloved Mini Cooper, nicknamed Enid.

My assessor was called Matt, a young guy who did rally driving/racing at weekends! I'm sure you need something like that if you spend your working life around disabled drivers.

The first couple of hours were spent drinking coffee and talking. Unfortunately the questionnaire I filled in never got to Matt so we went over this a little. Then he tested the strength of my upper body, which I knew was pretty good.

[1] No, please.

Then the embarrassing bit. He got me to push down with my feet and flex up again. I knew this wasn't going to be very good and sure enough, it was truly pathetic. Not surprisingly then, he declared that I needed hand-controls to drive. I'm sure you can imagine the pictures that went through my brain – a small, three-wheeler, light blue disabled car.

But I put on a brave face, and pushed these thoughts to the back of my mind, and concentrated on seeing Enid with additional hand controls. It'll be all right I told myself. Then the killer, it would have to be automatic. I tried to argue, but was told that my two remaining driving limbs, my hands/arms, would have too much to do to be able to change gears as well.

Bye-bye Enid.

Very sad. I was beginning to realise that my car was an important part of my self-image. So very, very sad.

Still, nobody had died and I decided to view the test drive with hand-controls as a challenge.

My contest with the hand-controlled car began after lunch. Actually, I was feeling pretty up-and-at 'em by then because I'd scored pretty well (above average, anyway) on the cognitive tests that Matt had done with me just before lunch. In fact, he said he'd never seen anyone answer a sorting test in the same way as I had done! (Was this good/bad? It certainly showed that my brain works in a strange way!)

Back to the hand-controlled car, a Ford Focus, much to my husband's delight. (He'd love to get me driving one of those!).

Matt drove us to a car park and then it was my turn to drive. To cut a long story (and many unsuccessful tours of the car park) short, I hated the hand-controls. It was so alien to normal driving (which I'd been doing[2] for thirty years) that it really addled my brain (and hands, and feet).

Matt called it a 'multi' something system – I guess because one stalk that stuck out from the bottom of the steering wheel did a multitude of tasks. You had to push it down to put the brakes on, pull it upward to accelerate and it also had the indicator as a switch on the same stalk. But, was this a self-cancelling indicator? Was it, hell. And you steered by having your left hand on a knob on the wheel.

So, imagine you're coming up to a left turning.

—You're slowing down (remember you've got to push the stalk <u>away</u> from you).

---

[2] Some would argue with the description of "normal". I even scared a driver who used to scare everyone else. Personally, I don't understand it – I thought I'd driven with him in a fairly restrained manner.

—On the same stalk, you need to indicate left (probably with your thumb).

—Keep slowing down (push away from you).

—Turn left (turn the wheel with your left hand only — remember your right hand is doing the braking and the indicating). Hope it's not a sharp turn or else your hands will get crossed over!

—When the car is straight, start to accelerate out of the corner (remember you've got to pull the stalk towards you).

—And, as quick as you can, turn off the indicator (same stalk), while still accelerating (pulling the stalk towards you).

And that's the easier direction. Imagine turning right!

At traffic lights!

I hated it! My feet tried really hard to help which is ironic since they've become pretty reluctant to do anything useful recently — hence the need for hand-controls.

Once we returned to HQ[3] with me driving, I was so tired[4] that I nearly decided to call it a day and not bother trying the other system. Fortunately, I kept my mouth shut and went on to try the other system.

You've probably guessed already that the "other" system was much, much better for me. It still had a lever to the right of the steering wheel that you push down for the brake, but that was the only purpose of this "stalk". That alone suited me more[5] — can't be doing with rehearsing a rhyme[6] to remember which way to push or pull the lever.

So, having chosen the system for me, Guido-Symplex by name, I agreed with Gary to come back for 10 one-hour lessons to learn how to use it.

Finally, after five hours (although this included 30 minutes for lunch)[7] at the centre in Welwyn, Alan took me home. Thank goodness.

Driving Lessons

This was a very odd experience after 30 years of driving.

Obviously, I'd picked up a few bad habits[8], but I like to think that this would apply to virtually everyone. I got used to the hand-controls fairly

---

[3] Yes, Matt did let me drive out on the open road using this multi-something set of controls. Fortunately he put an "L" plate on the roof of the car so other drivers would approach me with caution – very wise! I really needed their patience.

[4] And pissed off, I expect.

[5] One thing at a time, that's me. I remember my old boss once criticising me for only being able to do one thing at a time – just one research project at a time then, in amongst the personnel issues, the bookkeeping, invoicing and managing/writing the BS5750 document. Am I bitter? Yes, I am.

[6] OK, with the multi-system you push down to put on the brakes (slow down) and pull up to speed up. It didn't come naturally.

[7] Which we spent in the local supermarket car park eating some such cardboard food.

[8] Well, more than a few really.

quickly, although the car I was driving was a bit sluggish. This was another Ford Focus belonging to the centre[9].

Unfortunately the car, as well as being adapted with a Guido-Simplex system, had a big box, designed to take wheelchairs, on the roof. The problem was that the box made quite a lot of noise, especially around 40+mph. Since I've always driven according to the noise level a car makes,[10] I found it hard to go much above 40 on the MOTORWAY. I couldn't believe it – ME going very SLOWLY on the motorway. Of course, going so slowly was hazardous and I got tooted quite a lot.

Not only did I go too slowly on the motorway, I went too fast on the other roads. These, and other foibles, led to Matt being worried, even after 10 hours of lessons, about the way I drove, "You're a bit of a girl racer, aren't you?" On the one hand this was quite a compliment from a part-time rally driver, plus no-one had called me a "girl" for over quarter of a century. But Matt felt I'd failed the assessment that he did after these ten lessons and therefore thought I needed more lessons before I could be regarded as fit to drive. He reported this back to the DVLA.

So the DVLA have asked for me to be assessed again. I've arranged to be assessed at a different place – MAVIS, down in Crowthorne, Berks. I just don't want to go back to the same place where I failed before. I can also do the assessment in my own car, which has been adapted to the hand controls. It won't be until September, but hopefully I'll pass then.

I'm confident because I've been having lessons with an instructor who comes to me so that I don't have to travel. That makes me much more fresh when I drive and, with more practice, I think I drive better now that I've adapted my driving to a more sedate pace. This makes more sense since I've got 50% less limbs that I can use now. My instructor thinks I'm better too, so it's not just me!

It's also helped me enormously that I have replaced Enid with another car that I'm very happy with. This was very important to me – girl racer I may be, but a girl's got her image to think of! So, I bought a Mercedes SLK 230! I won't go into the machinations it took to persuade the car adapters that they could fit a Guido-Simplex system into a Mercedes, but they did – eventually.

It was worth the pain and the wait because I feel like a member of the human race again when I drive it. Occasionally I get beeped at by a motorist who expects me not to brake so early for a corner or to go faster generally.

---

[9] And yes, my husband was delighted again!
[10] And, you guessed it; it was my husband who pointed out this tendency of mine.

But I have to serenely ignore them because both of these are features of driving when you can only use half of your limbs. Since you have to use your right hand to brake, it leaves only your left hand to steer. So, it's better to finish with the braking before you get to the corner so that you've got both hands to steer. This is true for most corners. It's also true that it's better not to race around[11] generally, since you have less resources to draw upon if things go wrong, so having more time to spot and correct things must be a good idea.

---

[11] By this I mean sticking to the speed limit, including motorways!

FEELING REALLY ANGRY – A BAD FEW DAYS

Being Miserable

For the first time in all the 19 years since I was diagnosed, including the 6 years since I had to stop work, I am angry. I'm angry at everything. The whole world. And possibly worst of all, angry with myself.

How come this MS rubbish happened to me? How come someone, who had so much to give, got struck down like this? I was beginning to get somewhere with doing market research amongst kids and teenagers and it gave them a voice. The voice was well worth listening to, but I had to stop before it really got heard.

And I've never been angry before. Sad, yes. Feeling sorry for myself, yes. But never angry. Not like this.

This feeling hasn't been caused by one thing. It runs too deep for that. What happened?

- The improvements that happened to me while in Birmingham have disappeared. I believe I can get them back in the end, but it's a lot of hard work and I need more help.
- Not being able to drive a manual any more, knowing I'll never drive Enid again and having to use hand-controls, never pedals again, is a real blow. I know it's not the end of the world and as Boris Becker said once, having lost a major match at Wimbledon, "No one died," but it's simply not fair. To begin with I thought, "I'll make the best of this and have a convertible," but there is still a sense of loss – it wasn't my decision to sell the Mini – I just have to. I'm not a control freak (honest!) but I am angry.
- Not being able to do very much other than manage the house and all its contents (including furry occupants), makes me very sensitive to criticism. One of our cats had her back-quarters crawling with maggots the day after I expressed concern about her and thought she should go to the vet. I was over-ruled; "we take the cats to the vet too quickly", he said. You can imagine that made me angry, especially since she's really quite poorly now. The maggots have got a long way into her skin and she's really down. Nobody deserves that – at least I

haven't got maggots.

The picture below shows her once some of her fur has grown back. It's growing back grey – a designer cat!

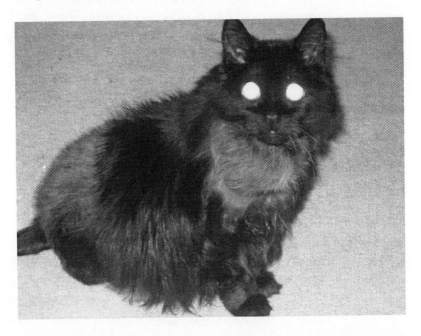

- Both Alice and Tom are away – a long way away – South Africa and India respectively. Not only do I miss them, they're such a tonic for me, but also their absence means there's no one that I have to be strong for. That contributes to the anger too because I'm missing two of the "stop" buttons that prevent the anger taking over.

Being Even More Miserable

I hate this fucking illness. I really, really do.

I've spent all day crying my heart out.

I thought if I spoke to my computer about it, I might get it out of my system and maybe feel a bit better.

I'm sick of it. I've lost sight of the things that I can still do. (Are there any?) All I can think about is the things that are going wrong – not just to or for me but I've got it into my head that it isn't too great for other people close to me, either.

Maybe it would be better if I just wasn't here. Then everyone could move on and not have to worry about or consider me. I've thought about suicide once before. Obviously I didn't do anything about it then.

And I guess I'm too much of a coward to do anything about it now. I really, really love my kids, and I don't want to leave them. Anyway, being selfish, I want to see what happens to them. I want to meet their partners and any children that they have.

But who wants a decrepit old granny around?

What Do You Want From Other People?

While I was in this black mood, a friend rung up and after I whittered for a while, asked me the question above. This was my answer.

Respect: to understand that while my body doesn't work very well, I'm not stupid. In fact I'm quite bright. No, not quite, very.

I'm still the same person that I used to be.

Appreciation: to appreciate what I can do – it's not as much as I used to do – but my brain still works – I can understand, think and decide. I'm not a prevaricator, nor do I procrastinate. My fingers work enough to use the phone and my computer. Plus I respect other people – I believe that everyone is human and has a right to be treated with respect. Basically, people tend to like me – if I ask for help they tend to provide it unhesitatingly. I don't mean helping me only in the practical sense, although I do need things doing for me, my kids, my pets and my home. My husband could do with practical help too, as well as time to relax and do 'his own thing'.

Recognition: I need to be recognised as a woman. I can't wear certain things any more – mainly on my feet – high, thin, sexy heels and pointed-toed shoes. I can't dance now – I tend to fall over – but I used to love it. In my time, I've stopped discos (clubs, to the offspring) stone dead, with people watching me (John Travolta – eat your heart out!) I can't 'bowl' people over any more – even the sexiest of dresses just doesn't look the same if you're in a wheelchair or, on better days, if you're walking with a stick.

Loving care: related to the above, sex is pretty important – nothing underlines disability more for me than the feeling that someone thinks you can't "do it" any more. Or that you're not interested any more. Or that you're not desirable any more.

Support: I mean emotional support. Understanding, empathy and optimism. I've got a very good friend, whom, although he has his down moments (fair enough) has an inherent brightness about him that does me a power of good. Contrast this with a husband who is incredibly negative, and who, at times, sits on my shoulders like a ton weight.

Reading this again, many times, I wonder what right I have to ask all this. I'm not perfect, I know. I'm too proud to ask for help very often. I'm too sensitive and I'm terrified of being rejected. I also hate being ignored. Am I difficult to live with, MS or no MS? Yes, I think so.

Did writing all this make me feel any better? I don't really know. I think I need to go and rest though. Bye.

Back Again

It's the next day now, and I've gone back to taking the Amantadine. The reason for this is that I got my husband to read the "side-effects" that my new drug, "Modafil," has. I didn't want to read them myself because I know I'm incredibly suggestible – so I never read about "side-effects" because I know I'll get them! I asked him to look out for references to "depression" in case this new drug was contributing to how shitty I've been feeling these past few days.

The list of "side-effects" was apparently long, but he managed to find a reference to depression. That's enough for me. Alan suggested that I go back to Amantadine today for a couple of days and see how I feel. I think I already feel a bit more positive and less inclined to feeling sorry for myself. The tendency for me to bite the head off anyone stupid enough to come near me has also mostly evaporated.

Going for a piss more often was also a side effect apparently (along with many others). That explains why I had to change my clothing three times the other day. Thankfully, that's stopped now too – it's still urgent[12] – but at least I'm in with a chance not to evacuate myself before I get to the loo

---

[12] Maybe a minute's warning which is enough if your legs work. But, if they don't – it's touch and go whether you get there in time

---

NEW THINGS ON THE HORIZON

More Recognition of Different Types of MS

I have written how, to a mere laywoman, more forms of MS seem to have been identified as the years have progressed. I recently read an article by Professor Alan Thompson, the MS Society's Medical Adviser, about Primary Progressive MS.[13] I think that finally, in the summer of 2005,[14] I recognise the type of MS that I have now, namely the Primary Progressive one.[15] Although maybe it was Benign to start with.

The descriptions that were key were:

- "In PPMS, the most fundamental difference is that people do not have relapses and remissions, which are generally seen as the defining features of MS."[16]
- "In around 80 to 90 per cent of people with PPMS, their MS mainly affects the spinal cord...."[17]
- ...they develop a stiffness and weakness of both legs"
- "....the condition continues in the same way as it begins....so the problem tends to be in one main area, often related to walking,
- though people may also experience bladder...dysfunction.[18]"

Apparently, PPMS only affects about 10% of people diagnosed with MS – I had to be one of them, didn't I?

Whether PPMS, which does not have relapses and remissions, ought to be diagnosed as a category of MS on its own is, however, a good question.

My humble answer, as someone with PPMS but not a medic, is yes – PPMS should be diagnosed as a separate category. The worry expressed in the article that this would "make (PPMS) people feel different and excluded from more 'mainstream' MS research" would, for me, be hugely outweighed by the feelings that

a) PPMS is being recognised and
b) that research may be more fruitful if subjects' type of MS was taken into account so that the data consisted of analysable 'type of MS' sub-groups[19].

---

[13] MSMATTERS 59 INSIGHT
[14] It only took twenty years then!
[15] Before, as I related in section 2, I thought it was 'Benign' because nothing really happened or changed in the first 13 years. Maybe both descriptions apply to me.
[16] That would explain why a lot of people to whom I mentioned I had MS referred to "good" days and "bad" days. It always puzzled me, but I didn't like to say anything, since it seemed good that people at least knew something about the condition.

Indeed, the article goes on to ask many questions that relate specifically to PPMS and says that finding answers to these would probably help other forms of MS. Producing information that is specific to PPMS would help people like me (and others) too, since apparently information about relapsing remitting MS does not apply to PPMS. More importantly, a better understanding of PPMS will hopefully lead to better treatment.

Goat Serum

Goat Serum, also known by its trade names of Aimspro and Caprivax, holds hope for MS sufferers

Improvements have apparently been reported in walking ability, bladder and bowel problems, strength, balance, fatigue, better control of fine movements, well being, feeling mentally more alert and more 'normal'. This list seems to include many of the symptoms that are problems for me.

To say that I can't wait to get my hands on it would be an understatement – I'm on a mission now to do just that. The idea that patients need to inject themselves once a week, probably for life, doesn't bother me at all, since I already do this with Beta Interferon.

At the moment, the only hope of receiving Aimspro is on an 'informed consent' basis. Upon making various phone calls, however, it appears that the few routes that were open are now closed. At least one trial appears to have stopped because the control sample (unknowingly receiving a placebo instead of Aimspro) were doing so much worse than the Aimspro sample, that it was deemed unethical to continue.

It is still unlikely to be less than 2 – 3 years before Aimspro becomes available. Apparently, that is still "quick" for a new drug.

I can only add my voice to that of the charity Proventus to try and speed up the trial results that are due now and expedite the process that could result in the drug becoming available.

I have written to the company, Daval International Ltd, asking to go on the 'Informed Consent' list – there's only over 2000 people ahead of me!

The latest I've heard, from Proventus[20], is that "Aimspro is not in production anywhere in the world" and "will not be produced anywhere until a specials license either in the UK or elsewhere is granted".

[17] My consultant had said that my spinal cord was mainly affected
[18] That's me too. Urgency and frequency (five times a night on bad nights) sums it up.
[19] Very recently, hearing Lee Dunster, Head of Research and Information at the MS Society, refer to results by type of MS was brilliant. It would be great to enhance this and encourage the media to differentiate more effectively between RR, SP and PP types of MS so that "MS research stories" become clearer
[20] On August 14, 2005

WHAT'S NEXT?

Well, I don't know.

I've got lots of things that I hope will happen, not just for me, but for everyone that I've whittered about and a few that have been spared.

Most of all I guess, I wish for a breakthrough in the treatment of MS, especially one that includes PPMS.

I know that I'm not alone in this, and if anybody thinks of anything I can do then please let me know.

And how do I feel having written this book? Well, I'm not sure. It started as a way of talking to myself, as a kind of therapy, I suppose. Then the odd person who read my outpourings found it interesting and thought that maybe others might benefit from it. Finally, it's prompted me to look around and find out more about the whole area.

In the end, I'm feeling quite sad. I wonder if we've become slaves to our scientific ideals. The medical profession demands 'evidence' – double blind controlled sample testing. I'm sure that this is with the very best of intentions; they don't want to build up hopes that then get shattered. Believe me, my friends, I can live with the gamut of emotions that I've been through. It's hardest to live with no hope.

An over-riding feeling of impotence is also a tough thing for me to deal with. I really, really would like at least some of my life back.

Reading this again it feels quite negative. This is the opposite of what I wanted to project which, overall, could be encompassed by the feeling, "Stay positive and laugh, or stay in the dark and die".

With this happy thought, I'll sign off with the idea of pursuing stem cell therapy. This is, of course, as advocated by Christopher Reeve after his horrendous riding accident and even George W had a thing or two (mainly negative) to say about it. The controversy was about using human foetal cells although, now I've had a chance to find out more[21], it appears that cells from the umbilical cord and placenta (once a baby has been born) can be used. I'm really excited about going to Holland to do this, particularly since there seems to be something, dare I say, magical about it. Not only due to the way it was brought to my attention, but also because the doctor I spoke to in Rotterdam believes Aqua Tilis Therapy and removal of amalgams are both beneficial precursors to stem cell treatment. Were the angels with me or not?